Reflections on Artificially Supplied Nutrition and Hydration

Proceedings of Quodlibet 2004

Contents

Introduction

With its continuing interest in the care of vulnerable patients and in promoting a culture of life, the Canadian Catholic Bioethics Institute organized its 2004 Quodlibet around the topic of the provision of artificially supplied nutrition and hydration. In this volume of *Proceedings* are the papers presented at that gathering and a culminating reflection statement on the issue.

The Quodlibet was held only months after the publication of Pope John Paul II's address, "To the Participants in the International Congress on 'Life-Sustaining Treatments and Vegetative State: Scientific Advances and Ethical Dilemmas' ". (We include the text of the statement starting on page 139 in this volume.) Professor Joseph Boyle's opening presentation, "Towards Ethical Guidelines for the Use of Artificial Nutrition and Hydration", provided a close examination of the papal text, working through nuances and suggesting how it might be interpreted and applied.

While the papal statement became an important reference point at the Quodlibet, discussions were not limited to the care of patients in a so-called persistent vegetative state. In his paper, "The Role of Artificial Nutrition and Hydration in the Care of the Frail Elderly: Empirical Issues and Disputed Questions", Dr. William Sullivan considered the issue as it pertained to the care of other vulnerable patients—the frail elderly, as well as patients suffering from strokes, neuro-degenerative conditions and terminal illnesses.

Other presenters covered different aspects of the issue. Drawing on precedents being set in Australia, Dr. Nicolas Tonti-Filippini presented his paper, "Advance Directives and Substitute Decision-Making in Relation to Providing Food and Water" which explored the challenges posed by advance directives and substitute decision-making around artificially supplied nutrition and hydration.

Rev. Kevin O'Rourke, meanwhile, provided a detailed examination of the foundational terms "ordinary" and "extraordinary" means, and of "terminal illness" and "fatal pathology" in his presentation, "Some Ethical Considerations Concerning Ordinary and Extraordinary Means to Prolong Life".

After spending their time at the Quodlibet in prayer and discussion, listening to papers and considering cases, participants then drew up a list of proposed guidelines, subsequently published in *The National Bioethics Quarterly* and included in this volume of *Proceedings*. The list of signatories attests to the commitment of the participants to a faith meant to be lived in-this-world—which is what it means to be called to be God's Kingdom on earth.

Many thanks to Leo Walsh, CSB, for his help in reviewing the papers contained in this volume of *Proceedings*. I am grateful as well to Bambi Rutledge and Jo-Anne Jackson-Thorne for their tireless and very fine work in preparing the manuscript.

Bridget Campion

Towards Ethical Guidelines for the Use of Artificial Nutrition and Hydration

Joseph Boyle

ANH is an acronym for "artificial or artificially provided nutrition and hydration". I take it that this expression refers to efforts of caregivers to provide nourishment and hydration to a person independently of that person's own activities of eating and drinking. ANH is used when a person cannot eat or drink or when a person's eating and drinking are in some way problematic as, for example, when efforts to feed the person orally are expensive or unsuccessful.

The widespread use of ANH for people in various conditions has raised ethical questions concerning the circumstances under which ANH should be used and not used, including situations which might warrant discontinuing the use of ANH, as conditions change after it was appropriately initiated. Clearly there is a need for guidelines to assist patients, families, health care and other helping professionals in addressing the moral complexities of this increasingly common intervention.

Joseph Boyle, PhD, is a Professor in the Department of Philosophy, University of St. Michael's College in the University of Toronto, Canada. This chapter was published with changes in Boyle, J., "Towards Ethical Guidelines for the Use of Artificial Nutrition and Hydration," in C. Tollefsen (ed) *Artificial Nutrition and Hydration: The New Catholic Debate*, Vol. 93, Philosophy and Medicine book series and no. 5 of the Catholic Studies in Bioethics subseries; Dordrecht: Springer 2007.

Different moral communities and traditions will approach the task of formulating such guidelines differently, drawing on resources of their traditions in various ways. The guidelines towards which this essay points are based on the Roman Catholic tradition.

The Catholic tradition has much guidance to offer health care decision-making, especially those decisions that may shorten a person's life or seriously affect his or her vocational commitments. That guidance is found in the principles and casuistry of Catholic moral teaching, and is sometimes addressed by popes and bishops in specific moral teaching.

In the case of the use of ANH, there is not only the traditional teaching about ordinary and extraordinary treatments and the complex teaching about euthanasia, but also a very recent papal teaching on the use of ANH for patients in what is somewhat unfortunately called "persistent vegetative state" (PVS).[1] Although the condition of persistent vegetative state occurs rarely, and although the features which make decisions about the use of ANH for patients in that condition are not common to most decisions about ANH, a careful look at the papal statement is a necessary step in the undertaking of formulating Catholic guidelines and a useful entry into that effort.

Pope John Paul II's Address on the Persistent Vegetative State

A brief, analytical summary

This address is a short speech made up of seven numbered paragraphs.

In the first paragraph, John Paul II greets the group of experts gathered by the Pontifical Council *Pro Vita* to discuss the ethical issues that arise in caring for patients in persistent vegetative state. He announces the focus of his talk: "the complex scientific, ethical, social and pastoral implications" of the condition of patients in PVS. So, the focus is PVS and not ANH except as used for those patients in this condition.

In the second paragraph, John Paul II explicitly outlines his understanding of the clinical and neurological aspects of PVS.

Drawing on the relevant clinical and scientific evidence, John Paul II defines the vegetative state as the absence of evident signs of self-awareness or of the environment, and the apparent inability to interact with others or to react to specific stimuli. He also underlines a morally important implication of the condition: those in it are completely dependent on others.

Before considering how the vegetative state comes to be defined "permanent" or "persistent", John Paul II reflects on the diagnosis and prognosis of the condition. Diagnosis is quite difficult, as the high number of reported diagnostic errors indicates. The prognosis for those given appropriate treatment and rehabilitation is mixed —some patients have emerged from the condition, but others remain in it "even for long stretches of time and without needing technological support." Later in this paragraph he suggests we lack the resources to distinguish patients having these very different prospects, even among those whose vegetative condition persists.

He next considers the persistence or permanence of the vegetative condition of some patients. A vegetative state is deemed to be "persistent" when it has continued for a year, a term chosen not because a medical factor could emerge within that time frame to change the diagnosis, but because of the fact that, as a matter of statistical summary, patients who remain in vegetative state for a year are very unlikely to recover from it. Furthermore, their chance of recovery gets progressively lower as time goes on. John Paul II notes, however, that even some patients who remain in a vegetative state for many years recover from the condition. He concludes that medical science cannot predict with certainty who, among patients in this condition, will recover and who will not.

In paragraph three, John Paul II states in general terms the Church's normative position on how people in this and other similar conditions of grave debility are to be treated. He begins by reflecting on the reference of the term "vegetative" in the widely used, but unfortunate, name for this condition. It is a term that refers not to the patient, who remains a human being, but to the clinical state. If taken as referring to the sick person as such, this expression actually demeans the person's value and personal dignity. This central affirmation is that a human being remains a human being as long as she or he is alive. However debilitated his or her condition: "I feel the duty to reaffirm strongly the intrinsic value and personal dignity do not change, no matter what the concrete circumstances of his or her life." This means that a person who is disabled in the exercise of higher human functions does not become an animal or a vegetable. So, human dignity remains for these people: "the loving gaze of God the Father continues to fall upon them, acknowledging them as his sons and daughters, especially in need of help."

In the fourth paragraph, John Paul II applies the general considerations in paragraph three to the clinical reality described in paragraph two. He first addresses the general rights of persons in PVS and then considers the specific issue of the use of ANH for these patients. The rights of these patients are correlative with duties of health care professionals, society and the Church, the non-fulfillment of which will lead to a failure of solidarity and of professional ethics.

He lists the rights of patients in PVS "awaiting recovery or a natural end": the right to basic health care, including such things as nutrition, hydration, warmth and cleanliness; the right to the prevention of complications related to confinement to bed; and the right to appropriate rehabilitative care and monitoring.

Turning to the use of ANH for these patients, and in particular to the decision to withdraw ANH, John Paul II begins with two distinct normative affirmations: first, the use of ANH for these patients is a natural means of preserving life and not a medical act. No explicit conclusion is drawn immediately, but the context suggests this is given as a reason for holding the continued use of ANH to be obligatory.

The second point is logically independent from the first, connected to it by the conjunctive "furthermore". It is that the use of ANH in such patients is "in principle ordinary and proportionate and as such morally obligatory, insofar as and until it has achieved its proper finality, which in the present case consists in providing nourishment to the patient and alleviation of his suffering."

He goes on in a statement that appears to draw together into a conclusion the two preceding points: normal care due to the sick in such cases includes the provision of hydration and nutrition. He then observes that this obligation of minimal care is not overridden by the judgement that recovery from PVS is very unlikely.

John Paul II then develops what appears to be an independent line of argumentation against withdrawing ANH from these patients: that if done on the basis of the dim prospects of recovery, it is a case of euthanasia by omission. He begins by noting that the inevitable outcome of withholding ANH from these patients is death by starvation or dehydration. He then notes that, if done knowingly and willingly, the decision to withhold ANH, presumably on the basis of this judgement about unlikely recovery, is euthanasia by omission.

He wraps up this central paragraph with a reminder that doubts about the presence of a human life are to be settled in favor of the life, and so the possible presence of human life precludes actions aiming at anticipating its death.

The fifth paragraph addresses the challenge posed by "quality of life" considerations, which John Paul II thinks are often dictated by outside psychological, social and economic pressures. He notes that such considerations cannot override the moral principles articulated and applied in paragraphs three and four. He spells out three specific implications of this general ethical observation: first, costs cannot outweigh the good of human life. Second, no external assessment of the quality of a person's life can be a ground for compromising human dignity. Any such ground introduces a discriminatory and eugenic principle into social relations. Third, the withdrawal of ANH might well cause patients in PVS much suffering.

In the sixth paragraph John Paul II affirms the social obligation to take positive steps to oppose the withdrawal of nutrition and hydration, especially by supporting the families of people in this condition. He takes note of the "heavy human, psychological and financial burden" borne by the families of those in PVS and concludes that support is necessary. Although the care of these patients is not, in general, particularly costly, society should make resources available for the care of this kind of frailty.

In the final paragraph John Paul II highlights his conclusion: the medical profession is "to cure if possible, always to care." He grounds this exhortation in the Lord's words, "Amen I say to you whatever you did to these least brothers of mine you did for me."

Some Comments

As his parting comments highlight, John Paul II thinks that the provision of ANH to patients in PVS is a requirement of normal care and is in this sense obligatory. He recognizes that this obligation can be onerous, at least for the families involved. He does not say, but natural law implies that the particular forms of the duty to care are inevitably limited by the responsible agent's capacity to provide care, not least by the other grave responsibilities the person may have. For some poor families without the third party support of socialized medicine or insurance, there might be very little they could afford by way of medical care for a debilitated family member. But that does not remove their duty to care; it changes its shape.

Likewise, the obligations of political society to guarantee support for people suffering various forms of grave debility and for their families are limited by other social responsibilities. Of course, the rationing of health care and of other resources in the world as it actually exists is a virtual necessity that will be morally proper only if it is done in accord with the principles of fairness. Those principles exclude putting a price on a human life, but they do not exclude using scarce resources for some and not for all who have need of them. And the Pope seems to be arguing that we will not treat fairly patients in PVS unless we continue to care for them and that includes maintaining the ANH that was in place as they developed this condition. So, it is morally significant that the costs of care for these patients are not high. For if they were, the requirements of fairness might be different and the form taken by the social duty to care might vary in ways similar to those in which an unsupported family's duty varies.

But plainly John Paul II thinks that there are other morally compelling considerations at play in these cases besides the requirements of social solidarity, namely, that providing ANH to these patients is in principle ordinary means and so obligatory, and that withdrawing it is at least sometimes euthanasia by omission.

I understand ordinary treatments to be those not involving grave burdens. Burdens are the bad side effects of treatment, understood broadly. If these are either insignificant or not sufficiently important to justify making their avoidance the basis for refusing the treatment, they are not grave. Extraordinary treatments, by contrast, are those having negative side effects so weighty that a person can reasonably choose to avoid those side effects, and so reasonably can decline the medical treatment. If a person chooses to reject ordinary treatments, that implies either that he or she is deliberately rejecting the good promised by the treatment, for example, continued life, or is insufficiently sensitive to the requirements of the good of life and health, perhaps from irrational fear of treatment or simple distaste for its rigors.

On this understanding of ordinary and extraordinary treatments, the nature of the standards for determining the bad side effects of the treatment to be gravely burdensome requires some articulation. I believe that the standard is ultimately the configuration of values and priorities set within a person's unique vocation. This standard allows for the wide diversity of judgements about what Catholic thought and practice accept as gravely burdensome without any suggestion that it is simply a matter of personal preference.

In the context of this brief account of ordinary and extraordinary means, John Paul II's judgement that providing ANH to patients in PVS is in principle ordinary treatment is intelligible. To consider such a question "in principle" seems to me to mean that the only factor about a patient's situation to be considered is the fact that he or she is in PVS, and the only aspect of care to be considered is the provision of ANH. Within this very specific context, to deem the provision of ANH to a patient in PVS "ordinary treatment" is to judge that the negative side effects of providing ANH to a person in PVS are not so serious as to justify withdrawing that treatment. Thus understood, John Paul II's judgement is clearly correct.

One reason for this is that providing ANH by a gastric tube seems to have relatively few negative side effects, especially for those patients in PVS, and even these side effects, we suppose, cannot be experienced by the patient. Moreover, as the Pope notes, the costs to the family, broadly construed, also seem generally low. And if there is a significant cost, it is the cost of the care as a whole and not of the ANH alone.

If John Paul II means something like this, his teaching does not exclude the possibility that there might be burdens sufficiently serious to justify abandoning the level of care that involves those burdens. However, abandoning a certain level of care— for example, in a hospital or nursing home because of a family's inability to pay—does not mean abandoning all care, and the need to move to a lesser level of care does not by itself justify withdrawing ANH. This is especially true if the reason to withdraw ANH is part of a decision to lower costs by ending the patient's life: costs go down because the patient dies, and stopping ANH contributes to the cost cutting because of its result in death. Hence the concern about euthanasia that John Paul II discusses.

Before turning to the issue of euthanasia, the condition John Paul II places on the obligation to continue ANH in these patients should be noted. He says this obligation holds "insofar as and until it is seen to have attained its proper finality, which in the present case consists in providing nourishment to the patient and alleviation of his suffering." Plainly this qualifier limits the obligation to cases where nourishment and alleviation of suffering are physically possible, and equally insists that ANH be provided when these ends can be met regardless of changes in the diagnostic situation. I do not think that John Paul II is overlooking the dynamism of the clinical and diagnostic situation, or rejecting the possibility of withdrawing a form of care such as ANH. He is suggesting, however, that, unless that dynamism reveals new or greater burdens that render the treatment gravely burdensome in changed circumstances, there will be a continuing duty to treat.

What precise connection does John Paul II make between the decision to withdraw ANH from a patient in PVS and euthanasia by omission? I take it that the idea of euthanasia by omission does not refer to all decisions to withdraw a treatment believed necessary for continued life (and so thought by the decision-makers sufficient or likely sufficient, given other causal factors already in play, to bring about death). For, plainly, many choices to forgo extraordinary treatments are of this kind. For instance, the choice to withdraw artificial respiration is often related to the patient's dying in exactly this way. Moreover, some actions that shorten life or inevitably lead to death are justifiable according to the principle of double effect.

Reflections on
Artificially Supplied Nutrition and Hydration

Proceedings of Quodlibet 2004
Toronto, Canada

Edited by
Bridget Campion, PhD

Canadian Catholic Bioethics Institute
Institut canadien catholique de bioéthique
Toronto

Thanks to Springer Academic Publishers for permission to reprint Boyle, J. (2007) "Towards Ethical Guidelines for the Use of Artificial Nutrition and Hydration," in C. Tollefsen (ed) *Artificial Nutrition and Hydration: The New Catholic Debate*, Vol. 93, Philosophy and Medicine book series and no. 5 of the Catholic Studies in Bioethics subseries. Dordrecht: Springer. ©Springer, with kind permission of Springer Science and Business Media.

Consensus Statement, "Reflections on Artificial Nutrition and Hydration: Colloquium of the Canadian Catholic Bioethics Institute (CCBI)" originally published in *The National Catholic Bioethics Quarterly*, 4:3 (Winter 2004), 773-782. © The National Catholic Bioethics Center. Permission to reprint granted: The National Catholic Bioethics Center, Philadelphia.

Address of John Paul II "To the participants in the International Congress on 'Life-Sustaining Treatments and Vegetative State: Scientific Advances and Ethical Dilemmas' ". Permission to reprint granted by the Libreria Editrice Vaticana.

Library and Archives Canada Cataloguing in Publication

Canadian Catholic Bioethics Institute. Quodlibet (2004 : University of St. Michael's College)
Reflections on artificially supplied nutrition and hydration : proceedings of Quodlibet, 2004 / edited by Bridget Campion.

ISBN 978-0-9731322-5-0

1. Artificial feeding--Moral and ethical aspects--Congresses.
2. Fluid therapy--Moral and ethical aspects--Congresses.
3. Medical care--Religious aspects--Catholic Church--Congresses.
4. Terminal care--Religious aspects--Catholic Church--Congresses.
5. Medical ethics--Religious aspects--Catholic Church--Congresses.
I. Campion, Bridget, 1955- II. Canadian Catholic Bioethics Institute
III. Title.

R726.C35 2009 179.7 C2007-905506-0

So, an intentional condition is required. The moral meaning of the choice not to do something or to stop doing something is specified by what goal that serves and by precisely how the choice to stop serves the goal. In euthanasia, the aim is to stop the patient's suffering by ending the patient's life. So, euthanasia by omission is a choice to stop a life-sustaining or life-extending treatment so that the person dies and suffers no more. If John Paul II is employing this understanding of euthanasia by omission, one can then see how withdrawing ANH from those patients in PVS can be euthanasia by omission. I suggested a version of this above, where death is chosen as a means to end expensive and burdensome care, and the withdrawal of ANH is the means to ending life. But John Paul II may be read as saying that any choice to withdraw ANH from a person in PVS is euthanasia. I suggest that this is a misreading.

As I have already suggested, euthanasia by omission is not any withdrawal of treatment that leads inevitably to death, but withdrawal or refusal of treatment involving the intention to end life for the sake of ending life. The rationale that John Paul II has in his sights here is that founded on the dismal prospects for recovery of a person in PVS. Implementing that rationale by a decision to withdraw ANH is difficult to formulate without including the patient's death as part of the plan. But what is it that practically connects concerns about these dim future prospects and a choice to end ANH? The patient in PVS is unlikely to recover, but continues to live. That condition is taken as bad, as indeed it is.

One way to put an end to the bad condition is to put an end to the patient's life: withdrawing ANH virtually guarantees that. If ANH is withdrawn to end the patient's life and so to put an end to a dismal condition with no prospect of recovery, then the choice to stop ANH is, if not euthanasia strictly speaking, then intentional homicide by omission. But plainly, this is not the only possible rationale for discontinuing ANH. Nevertheless, although I do not think that the Pope should be understood as holding that the withdrawing of ANH from those patients in PVS, is as such, euthanasia by omission (as it is in principle ordinary treatment), two quite common motivations for withdrawing ANH from those patients in PVS do involve a homicidal intent: namely, getting the treatment or the care over with, and avoiding the repugnant condition of life without recovery.

But it may seem that the life of such a patient is more than simply repugnant; it is somehow intolerable. Preserving such a life and caring for a person in that condition can seem worse than meaningless; it can appear to be an absurd suffering imposed on caregivers by a moral logic that has become divorced from reality.

The Pope plainly recognizes the real tragedy of those in PVS and the real burdens of those who care for them. But I think he would resist the idea that caring for those in PVS is absurd suffering. Our way of participating in God's loving providence is by pursuing the human goods according to the light of the principles of the natural law. That is what we have to guide our lives; not the full story of God's providence, but just what we must have to participate in God's plan as rational creatures. If we make good choices, then we have done our part. And if those choices involve actions that are deeply unsatisfying and troubling, the suffering that ensues is not absurd but justified, though we can only trust that the justification is there. Sometimes we get a hunch or are given a glimpse of that justification, but, for many of us much of the time, this kind of suffering leads to a terrible slog that faith alone can sustain as we try to do what is right.

Keeping people alive who likely will never again experience, think or interact with others seems absurd to many people, but it is not absurd if we think we cannot stop this effort without treating them unfairly, or without breaking faith with them, or even without intentionally ending their lives. The goods realized by refusing these choices are real, and even in our suffering we can experience them. And if the only way we can see through such situations is to do what continues our suffering, we must accept it.

What Guidance Does the Papal Statement on PVS Provide for Other Decisions about ANH?

I have emphasized in my exposition of and comments on John Paul II's address that his focus is primarily on the care of those patients in PVS, and not on ANH as such. I also emphasized that much of the moral vocabulary used by John Paul II is context and circumstance sensitive. What is part of the normal care that everyone is entitled to receive must vary as the capacities of providers and their social supports vary. What is ordinary treatment often does not emerge in the abstract description of a condition and its treatment, but becomes apparent only in circumstances that do not distinguish acts into generally described kinds. And the rationales in which the intentions of actions and omissions are revealed can vary considerably, even though the decisions themselves may appear to be clinically identical.

This suggests that the papal statement contains principles and patterns of moral reasoning that are widely applicable to decisions about ANH. There may be a more direct application of the papal teaching to decisions about the use of ANH in patients not in PVS. Certainly, in cases that are quite similar to PVS in their morally relevant features, the Pope's conclusions directly apply. In particular, in cases where the patient is not dying as long as ANH and comfort care are provided, but where the patient is not capable of conscious interaction with the environment and where recovery from that condition is most unlikely, then the papal teaching about PVS fully applies. For example, if those patients with Pick's disease[2] are for a time in a PVS-like condition, then removing ANH would be excluded, taking into account the traditional provisos I mentioned in the preceding section. But many of the choices about the use of ANH concern patients who are not unconscious, or whose prospects of recovery are real, or who may be able to swallow on their own, or who are so far along in the dying process that the benefit of extending life by ANH is so slight that, if they were assessed with a realistic acceptance of impending death, then ANH would not be used.

For example, the use of ANH to assist people in various conditions of dementia seems quite different from its use for those in PVS. Perhaps these people can eat and drink. If so, deciding to stop or not to start ANH for which there are medical indications, is not potentially euthanasia by omission. Moreover, there may be concerns that could make ANH contraindicated for these patients. There is evidence of increased morbidity and mortality caused by the use of gastric tubes, for instance. As well, because these patients can experience the intrusive effects of ANH, they may manifest a level of distress that, in the judgement of others, constitutes grave burden. So here, even if ANH is considered part of normal care, it must be assessed in terms of the burdens and benefits analysis of the ordinary/extraordinary means doctrine.

My conclusion is that the specific papal teaching about withdrawing ANH from patients in PVS is not readily exportable, and that it certainly does not exclude all choices to withhold or withdraw ANH. What are exportable, and should underlie any Catholic guidelines on ANH, are the principles that underlie the papal teaching. The most important of these has application far beyond the care for people in PVS, namely, the principle of human dignity that requires respect for the human person and insists that all human beings, however debilitated, are human persons.

This general principle has three more specific implications that are widely applicable to decisions concerning ANH:

> 1. a principle of solidarity or care for others, that challenges us to reach out to those most in need and to be fair-minded in our attitudes and use of resources for the benefit of the most disabled;
>
> 2. the doctrine of ordinary and extraordinary treatments that reminds us that the duty to act for our own and others' life and health is serious but defensible in the face of other grave obligations, especially those obligations that arise from each person's unique personal vocation; and
>
> 3. the absolute prohibition of deliberately choosing to end human life by act or omission for any reason whatsoever, however beneficent that reason may be. This norm is not self-applying, especially in the case of choices to refrain from or stop doing something that has some human point, since behaviorally similar choices not to do something can be very different moral acts depending upon one's reason for choosing.

In any human community shaped by what John Paul II has called the "culture of life", these three implications of human dignity will play an irreducible role. I suggest that they are a necessary ingredient in any set of guidelines for such a community. But none is a simple rule; each requires moral thinking and sometimes difficult moral analysis. I do not think that a set of guidelines made of easy-to-understand rules can capture this moral reality.

The Role of Advance Directives in Decisions Concerning ANH

The right of competent patients to refuse health care is widely accepted in modern societies. The extension of that right into the future to settle treatment issues that might arise after that person becomes unable to make decisions has also become widely accepted in the form of living wills and the appointment of proxies who have power to make decisions on the patient's behalf. Since this right and its extension have become part of the social fabric of modern health care, guidelines concerning decisions to use, decline, or stop using ANH must address the role of advance directives.

To begin I will give a very brief rationale for the right to refuse medical treatment and for its extension in advance directives. This rationale is not the popular secular argument which understands autonomy as an overriding value in health care and interprets it as implying that patients' desires establish what is right and wrong. Rather, it is an argument to the effect that the right of a competent person to refuse medical treatment is a generally reasonable allocation of decision-making authority in the social realm of heath care. The patient must live with the regimen of treatment and its consequences; they affect his or her vocation and life prospects most immediately. Health care professionals are not so directly affected and they are not public authorities but providers of expert advice and assistance. Such considerations as these seem to me to underlie older views about the right of competent patients to refuse treatment, the sort of views held by Pius XII, for example.

The idea of social authority is that, when there is disagreement about common action, which can happen in these decisions, someone must have the final say, and that person in the health care setting is most reasonably the patient him or herself. This understanding of decision-making authority does not imply that the patient's views are sound or altogether morally upright — only that they will prevail if there is disagreement. This is hardly patient autonomy in the modern sense.

If this right is accepted, then its extension by devices such as designating someone with power of attorney with respect to one's health care is also reasonable since one may, when unable to decide for oneself, face health care prospects in which one might be required to suffer unreasonably, or to impose on others in ways one can reasonably reject, or to use one's own or other's resources in ways one would prefer to avoid.

If this rationale for the right to refuse treatment is correct, then advance directives are a reasonable device. The question that arises in respect to ANH is whether any antecedent refusal of continued ANH must necessarily be a refusal of ordinary treatment or is conditional suicide by omission.

I think that the rationale for an advance directive, even including the refusal of such things as ANH if one were in PVS, need not be suicidal and could indeed be a completely virtuous and generous decision to free caregivers from their duty to use their time and resources to provide one with life-sustaining care. "Use your time, money and energy for other good things rather than keeping me going" is not necessarily suicidal, but can instead be a choice not to accept certain side effects of treatment – the costs in this case, of continuing treatment. By the vocational standard of seriousness

I suggested above, these side effects could reasonably be judged grave enough to justify forgoing them.

Of course, in our social environment, an advance directive to discontinue substantial elements of life-extending care such as ANH in conditions of great debility where prospects of significant recovery are lacking is likely to be based on a rejection of living in that repugnant condition. That would be suicidal.

If cooperating with what was surely a decision of this kind were necessarily formal cooperation, then cooperators would be guilty of willing suicide. However, respecting the social reality of the right to refuse treatment and its extension in advance directives does not involve intending the evils of those who misuse their authority to decide about their health care. And within a pro-life community, the presumption should not exist that instructed people will be guilty of conditional suicide.

In short, I think advance directives may rightly be used to deal with many aspects of medical treatment and care anticipated for future times when one is not competent to make decisions. Such directives can be abused and, when they certainly are being abused, those who respect human dignity will cooperate as little as possible with them. But when thoughtfully made, they can introduce moral wisdom into situations in which family and friends may need some help.

Notes

1 Pope John Paul II. Address of John Paul II "To the Participants in the International Congress on 'Life-Sustaining Treatments and Vegetative State: Scientific Advances and Ethical Dilemmas' " March 20, 2004. http://www.vatican.va/holy_father/john_paul_ii/speeches/2004/march/documents/hf_jp-ii_spe_20040320-congress-fiame_en.html. Reprinted with permission. See page 139.

2 Frontotemporal Dementia (also known as Pick's Disease) is a progressive dementia that affects the frontal and temporal lobes of the brain. The brain cells in these areas can shrink or die causing changes to behaviour and language skills. As the disease progresses, patients begin to present signs of dementia (forgetfulness and confusion) and loss of motor skills that may include difficulty in swallowing. http://www.alzheimer.ca/english/disease/dementias-frontotemp.htm (accessed March 10, 2007).

The Role of Artificial Nutrition and Hydration in the Care of the Frail Elderly: Empirical Issues and Disputed Questions

William F. Sullivan

In their commentary on a study by Callahan and colleagues that addressed the clinical question of the benefits for patients who underwent tube feeding, Thomas Finucane and Colleen Christmas conclude:

> On the one hand, [tube feeding] is a burdensome intervention of unproven benefit, and there is little justification for its use. On the other, it is a fairly non-invasive, arguably comfortable means of delivering nutrition and hydration to patients who are having difficulty eating, and it almost surely benefits some of these. We tend to take the former view, while Callahan and colleagues seem to tend toward the latter.... The paper by Callahan and colleagues is an important addition to the data that we should present to the decision-makers: "We do not have any information that makes us think your loved one will live longer or be more comfortable or functional if we do this procedure. We do know that if the PEG [Percutaneous Endoscopic

William F. Sullivan, MD, CCFP, PhD, is a Family Physician at St. Michael's Hospital and Surrey Place Centre and an Assistant Professor, Department of Community and Family Medicine, University of Toronto, Canada.

> Gastrostomy feeding tube] is placed, there is a very high chance that he/she will die soon."[1]

This commentary shows that both authors appeal to empirical data but draw opposite conclusions about the benefits and burdens of tube feeding or *artificial nutrition and hydration* (ANH). In developing ethical guidelines for ANH for the frail elderly with common medical conditions, it is important to review the medical literature, while being aware of the limitations of our current state of knowledge. For instance, there are no randomized trials comparing similar patients in terms of overall survival or tendency to aspirate, i.e., take fluids or solids into the lungs that could lead to pneumonia. Non-randomized studies show that patients with feeding tubes are not more likely to survive and are more likely to aspirate than patients without feeding tubes. These studies are informative so long as we understand that there may be factors other than the presence or absence of feeding tubes that account for the observed results. It is important to avoid either overly rash or overly hesitant conclusions based on the evidence provided by these studies.

This paper will review the current medical literature on ANH. My aim is to clarify current usage of medical terminology and the range of distinct medical conditions in which ANH is used. I will also try to synthesize some published empirical data on diagnostic or prognostic issues that might influence decisions about ANH and to evaluate the extent to which firm conclusions can be drawn. In some cases, these data will be helpful for the ethical debate and, in other cases, it will become evident that there are more fundamental issues that cannot be settled by further appeals to empirical data.

The Vegetative State/Post-Coma Unresponsiveness

The focus of the current debate over the use of ANH is on people with a neurological injury commonly known as a *Persistent* or Permanent Vegetative State (PVS). This controversy was addressed in a speech by John Paul II on March 20, 2004, "To the Participants in the International Congress on 'Life-Sustaining Treatments and Vegetative State: Scientific Advances and Ethics Dilemmas'," which outlined the principles at issue and their application to these cases.[2] In order to develop practical guidelines on the use of ANH generally, the focus of the discussion needs to be broadened to include more common medical conditions. It is estimated that among people receiving ANH, fewer than 1% are unconscious and even fewer are patients in a PVS. It is important, however, to examine some clinical issues and confusions that have arisen concerning PVS before discussing other, more common, medical conditions.

Classification

Vegetative state (VS) refers to the diagnostic category that Jennett and Plum defined in 1972 and refers to people with an unusual form of impaired consciousness.[3] In this condition, certain functions of the autonomic nervous system (previously referred to as the "vegetative system") are retained despite an unawareness of self and environment.[4] These patients may exhibit sleep-wake cycles in which they periodically open their eyes (unlike people in a coma). Also, they have retained sufficient hypothalamic and brain-stem function to maintain their respiratory and circulatory systems, so that these systems do not need to be supported by medical technologies such as a respirator, or medications to maintain blood pressure. However, these individuals show no evidence of responsiveness to the environment, nor of purposeful responses to stimuli, nor of language comprehension or expression.

A synonym for vegetative state recently recommended in an Information Paper produced by the government of Australia is *post-coma unresponsiveness* (PCU).[5] This latter term identifies a more restricted set of patients in whom the vegetative state follows from a severe brain injury that results in an initial period of coma. This diagnostic category excludes cases in which the vegetative state is the result of a congenital disorder, such as anencephaly, or is of a degenerative neurological condition that did not progress to a coma, such as advanced dementia. The prevalence of PCU in patients in the U.S. is estimated at between 15,000 and 35,000 at any given time or about 60 - 100 per million population (corresponding to 1,500 to 3,500 individuals in Canada).[6]

It is helpful to distinguish PCU from other types of impaired consciousness. *Consciousness* involves two essential components: wakefulness and awareness.[7] Persons in a *coma* are neither awake nor aware. Persons with *post-coma unresponsiveness* are awake but not aware. Persons in a state of *limited* or *minimal responsiveness* are awake and have some level of awareness. *Brain death* means that a person: (1) is unresponsive to external stimuli; (2) exhibits no evidence of brain-stem functions including spontaneous respiration and motor reflexes; and (3) this functional loss is irreversible.

Diagnosis

No single diagnostic radiological or laboratory test can confirm PCU. Hence, this condition is diagnosed mainly on clinical grounds, and the diagnosis is confirmed when the relevant clinical signs have persisted for one month.[8] Newer radiological techniques, such as *Positron Emission Tomography* (PET) scans, can demonstrate very low metabolic brain activity characteristic of vegetative states. However, such tests are not widely available. Although PCU is conceptually well-defined, even when the clinical diagnostic criteria are correctly understood and applied, it may be difficult to verify the diagnosis and distinguish PCU from minimally conscious states in which an aware patient cannot communicate.

Some contrary views have been expressed in the literature on both the diagnostic certainty of clinician judgements regarding PCU and the conceptual basis for this diagnostic category. First, rates of misdiagnosis of PCU reported in the literature are significant and range from 18% - 43%. These errors have been attributed to factors such as the type and frequency of assessments, the skills and experience of the assessor, and the more or less optimal conditions for patient assessments.[9]

However, there is speculation and some evidence that newer assessment tools and functional brain imaging techniques may increase the accuracy of these diagnoses and uncover a level of neurological function, possibly linked to awareness, that was previously undetectable. For instance, N400 brain waves have been detected in unconscious subjects in response to grammatically correct but semantically faulty sentences. As well, improved communication techniques have detected responsiveness in patients previously thought to be unresponsive.

There are philosophical objections to the diagnosis of PCU. Some argue that the determination of lack of awareness rests on the positivist presumption that consciousness or awareness exists if, and only if, it can be detected empirically. One criticism is that our empirical tools may be insufficiently sensitive to detect evidence of awareness. Another criticism is that the diagnostic criteria for PCU reduce properties of the mind to properties of the brain - a philosophically materialistic view of the human person. If one is not a materialist, one might not necessarily agree that empirical data are sufficient to rule out consciousness.

Prognosis

Leaving aside the controversy over the diagnosis of PCU, it should be noted that the prognosis for a coma is good. It is rarely permanent and typically lasts from hours up to four weeks. By contrast, when a coma evolves into an awake but unresponsive state, the prognosis for recovery is very low. Recovery depends on factors such as the cause of the brain injury, the duration of PCU, and the age of the patient. It is generally considered that, at six months in PCU following a brain injury from the lack of oxygen and twelve months in PCU following a traumatic brain injury, the probability of recovery is so low that the prognosis is described as "permanent". This means that, after a certain time, "a physician can tell the patient's family...with a high degree of medical certainty, that there is no further hope for recovery of consciousness [awareness] or that, if consciousness were recovered, the patient would be left severely disabled."[10]

The life expectancy for otherwise healthy patients in PCU is between two and five years. Death usually occurs as a result of related complications, such as respiratory infections, or from medical conditions that existed prior to coma, such as cerebro-vascular or coronary artery disease in the elderly. There are well known cases of younger people, however, continuing in PCU for decades.

Some contrary views on prognostic judgements for vegetative state (VS) have also been expressed in the literature. First, it is possible that a degree of uncertainty with regard to recoverability is an inherent feature of VS. When Jennett and Plum first discussed the prognosis of VS, they assumed that the prognosis of "permanent" would eventually be established statistically. They did not anticipate the possibility that uncertainty about recovering from VS might persist, nor that improvements in treatments might alter prognosis in certain cases.[11] The literature gives some evidence to support these possibilities. It appears that, for many, being conscious but severely disabled does not count as "recovery".[12]

It has also been pointed out that a prognosis of "permanent" qualifies but adds nothing new to the diagnosis of VS.[13] This prognostic judgement is usually not based on some new predictive neurological finding that has been identified in a particular patient. Rather, it is merely a matter of convention that those who are in PCU longer are more likely to continue in this state.[14]

Implications for Care

Persons with PCU are totally dependent on others for all of their care. Although they are capable of swallowing reflexively, they are unable to drink fluids or eat food orally. They will also require ongoing assistance with bladder and bowel functions, attention to skin and mouth health, and physiotherapy to avoid joint contractures.

Persons with correctly diagnosed PCU are incapable of "experiencing" in a way that a conscious subject would. Although some thinkers have argued that people in a PCU do suffer even if they are unaware of their condition, to the extent that consciousness is a necessary condition for personal suffering, these individuals cannot be said to suffer physically or mentally. Nor are they "subjects" capable of any cognitive acts, such as experiencing, understanding or judging.

Finally, since the underlying neurological condition of PCU is normally non-progressive, depending on the age, pre-morbid condition, and the level of care these patients receive, they may continue to live in this state for months, years, or even decades.

Questions

Despite the controversies regarding the diagnosis and prognosis of people in a state of post-coma unresponsiveness, there are two main questions that the literature addresses. First, can people be correctly diagnosed with post-coma unresponsiveness? Despite the high rate of diagnostic errors and the inability to confirm a complete lack of awareness, a correct diagnosis that distinguishes PCU from other states of minimal awareness seems possible most of the time. Second, is a prognostic judgement that this state is irrecoverable ever warranted? One may conclude that the recovery of consciousness (with or without disability) is very unlikely after a certain period of time, even though it is not impossible. Still, after a certain period of time in a PCU state, the probability of any recovery is statistically very small.

A key question for further consideration regards the goal and function of these diagnostic and prognostic labels. Do they really just function as a quality-of-life threshold? That is, are they helpful in classifying individuals who have similar levels of function and needs, so that they can be studied and their needs be better addressed? Or do these diagnostic and prognostic categories function merely to identify those who fall below a given level of cognitive function with no hope of "meaningful" recovery, and therefore determine the treatment or care that may or may not be offered to these patients? In other words, is the benefit/burden calculus regarding the use of ANH for patients in PCU any different from a quality-of-life determination?

Other Conditions in which ANH is Frequently Used

Does PCU, which represents a very small fraction (<1%) of cases in which ANH is provided, offer a useful paradigm for thinking about ANH in other more commonly encountered conditions (>99% of cases)? Do congenital and acquired pediatric disorders, various types of swallowing problems due to strokes or neuro-degenerative conditions in adults, and the final stages of dementia or a terminal illness raise different issues than PCU concerning the use of ANH? I will review briefly some of the clinical features of these different conditions. In a subsequent section, I will address the question of the morally relevant dissimilarities among these conditions to PCU that will need to be considered when formulating guidelines on the use of ANH.

Infants and Children with Cerebral Palsy

Children younger than 20 years old represent 6% to 38% of individuals in a VS (including those with PCU).[15] Of these, 41% may have had such congenital developmental malformations as anencephaly, 28% non-traumatic anoxia, and 21% traumatic brain injuries.[16] The most common type of brain injury for which ANH is used in children is *Cerebral Palsy* (CP). CP is "a non-progressive disorder of motion and posture due to brain dysfunction occurring before twelve months of age with commonly associated sensory and cognitive impairments."[17] Nutritional supplements delivered via feeding tubes are often provided temporarily for infants with CP until their oral intake of food is adequate. In some cases, ANH is provided on an ongoing basis.

Guidelines in pediatrics generally support the use of ANH in CP, but there have been no randomized studies in this area. Many clinicians are reportedly uncomfortable about forgoing ANH for their pediatric patients. They seem to regard the feeding of children as the most basic aspect of care. The extent of the infant's eventual neurological deficit cannot be known for certain in the first twelve months of life when decisions about providing ANH in CP commonly are made. ANH is seldom withdrawn from infants at a later point if it is life sustaining.

Cerebro-Vascular Accidents or Strokes

In Canada, the most common primary diagnoses among elderly adults receiving ANH are cerebro-vascular accidents or strokes (vs. dementia in the U.S.).[18] In contrast to patients with PCU, the vast majority of those with strokes (98%) are conscious and able to eat or drink to some extent, even if they have swallowing problems. Feeding issues relate primarily to dysphagia without mechanical obstruction and, secondarily, to insufficient nutritional intake. Dysphagia without obstruction can result in choking and, if severe and chronic, can cause patients to aspirate food and fluids into their lungs, resulting in pneumonia and possibly death.[19] Some authors argue that, with proper assessment and assistance in eating appropriate foods and liquids, many such swallowing difficulties can be adequately addressed without resorting to ANH by feeding tubes.[20] There is evidence that stroke patients with swallowing problems may recover better and more quickly if a feeding tube is placed early after the stroke rather than if it is placed several weeks later.[21]

A large study in the U.K. indicated that about a third of patients with strokes develop dysphagia and that, in a small percentage of these patients (1.7%), dysphagia persists beyond one month. These patients can, however, maintain adequate nutrition at home by means of a feeding tube. This study found that one year after this group started tube feeding at home, half continued, about a third had died, and the remaining patients (13%) had recovered their swallowing function and returned to normal eating and drinking. Patients seemed to be satisfied with tube feeding. Of those who were offered home tube feeding, very few refused (0.3%) or subsequently declined to continue (<1%). Moreover, the complication rate among stroke patients on home tube feeding was very low. Less than 1% required hospital admission for a complication within the first year of tube feeding.[22]

Neuro-Degenerative Conditions

The second most common group of individuals requiring ANH are those with various neuro-degenerative disorders. Although the most common neuro-degenerative disorder is dementia, ANH is also used for disorders that primarily affect motor rather than cognitive functions. These conditions include Amyotrophic Lateral Sclerosis and Parkinson's Disease, conditions that are progressive and incurable.

Amyotrophic Lateral Sclerosis (ALS) exclusively affects the motor system. It is characterized by a progressive loss of motor functions causing paralysis of muscles without the loss of sensory or cognitive functions. It usually begins by affecting distal muscles of the legs and gradually progresses towards the head by affecting neurons that control the muscles needed to cough and swallow. ANH sometimes plays a role in maintaining nutrition and alleviating swallowing difficulties, thereby reducing the occurrence of choking spells and the aspiration of food or fluids into the lungs. In ALS, some evidence supports the claim that ANH also prolongs life, particularly in those patients in whom swallowing symptoms occur near the onset of this disease. In ALS, death usually results from aspiration pneumonia. Since ALS only compromises motor functions, these patients are usually able to take part in decisions about their own care, including the use of feeding tubes and respirators.[23]

Parkinson's Disease (PD) primarily affects the motor functions. It is characterized by a rest tremor, increased muscle tone and a shuffling gait. These motor symptoms affect the coordination of muscle function needed to bring food to the mouth, chew and swallow safely. Significant feeding problems tend to occur late in PD when there may also be cognitive impairment that precludes patient involvement in decisions about feeding tubes. Symptoms of PD may also accompany other forms of dementia. Feeding tubes in patients with PD can be used mainly as a mode of delivering pills to those patients who have swallowing difficulties. Such medication may enable a patient with Parkinson's Disease to control his or her motor symptoms sufficiently to maintain oral nutrition. As in ALS, death most commonly occurs as a result of aspiration pneumonia.

Dementia primarily affects cognitive functioning, beginning with an irreversible loss of short-term memory. Age is the most important risk factor for dementia, and the number of people with dementia doubles every five years after age 65. A conservative estimate is that there are about four million people with dementia in the U.S. *Alzheimer's Disease* (AD) accounts for about 60% of cases of dementia in the elderly. *Vascular Dementia* (VD), which is caused by small strokes, is the second most common cause of dementia, accounting for between 10% to 25% of cases. Most patients with dementia are institutionalized four to six years after symptom onset, and spend three to four years in a nursing home before death.[24]

Disease progression is gradual and continuous in AD. By contrast, VD has an abrupt onset and stepwise progression with discrete episodes of decline following each small stroke.[25] The onset of AD may occur as early as forty years of age in certain genetically inherited forms. The course of AD can vary from five to twenty years. Early signs of AD include forgetfulness and loss of concentration. In more advanced stages, symptoms include language deterioration, impaired ability to manipulate visual information, poor judgement, confusion, restlessness, and mood swings. In the final stages of dementia, patients have profound impairments of cognition, personality and ability to function.[26] Medication may keep symptoms from becoming worse for a limited time. Patients most commonly die from infections. In the advanced stages, patients typically are unable to walk and feed themselves, are incontinent, and cannot recognize and communicate with people. It is normally during the advanced stages that feeding issues arise.[27]

The prevalence of tube-fed older residents of nursing homes in the U.S. is about 10%, of which about 60% have some form of dementia. There are institutional reasons for providing feeding tubes to these patients. Sometimes there are economic incentives for nursing homes to provide feeding tubes to residents. Feeding tubes may save staff time required to feed these patients by hand, and the institution may be paid higher premiums for caring for patients receiving tube feeding. Some institutions will accept patients with a swallowing problem only if they have a feeding tube. Alternatively, some nursing homes, especially in Ontario where nursing homes are distinct from long-term care facilities, will not accept patients with feeding tubes.

The purported medical benefits of tube feeding patients with dementia include preventing aspiration pneumonia, prolonging survival, reducing the risk of pressure sores, improving function and/or providing palliation. Some data suggest that tube feeding does not meet the expectations of prolonging survival, or of preventing aspiration pneumonia and pressure sores.[28] Finucane et al., however, found no published randomized controlled trials, the most strictly controlled type of research, that compared tube feeding with oral feeding in the elderly with dementia.[29] Hence, no definitive conclusion can be drawn.

The risks and burdens to the patient of tube feeding may not be trivial. One particular burden for individuals with dementia is the need for physical or chemical restraints in order to prevent them from pulling feeding tubes out. This often precludes the use of nasogastric tubes in patients with dementia, since these tubes are very obvious and irritating to patients. Hand restraints are likely to be needed during the first two weeks after gastrostomy-tube placement when it is important that the tube not be disturbed. After this initial period, patients are less likely to pull at their tubes and extubation is less problematic.[30] An alternative to ANH in those patients who can take some food and fluids by mouth is a program of hand feeding. If this fails, some guidelines suggest that ANH be tried with the consent of substitute decision-makers, who should be informed about its likely benefits and burdens.[31]

Cancer and Terminal Illnesses

Cancer is the second leading cause of death in most developed countries.[32] In the U.S., it is the third most common diagnosis among individuals receiving ANH. In cancers of the head and neck, a feeding tube may be used to bypass cancer related pharyngeal obstructions. It may also be used to allow adequate feeding around the times of major surgery, chemo or radiation therapy when the urge to eat is reduced or the ability to chew, swallow, retain and absorb food is impaired.[33] Some studies show that supported nutrition by tube feeding can improve the quality of life of patients with head and neck cancers when undergoing radiotherapy, as compared to those who continue on oral feedings. Patients in the former group were able to maintain their quality of life from a nutritional point of view, while those receiving oral feeding rapidly declined.[34]

In guidelines on ANH, cancer patients suffering from malnutrition have been categorized according to considerations such as the type of cancer and its extent as well as the likelihood of responding to treatment. If the cancer is incurable, the extent of the functional impact of the cancer and the patient's prognosis or proximity to death become important considerations. For example, one group of cancer patients consists of those who are undergoing therapy with a reasonable expectation of response or who are expected to live more than six months. Another group consists of malnourished cancer patients for whom treatments have been unsuccessful or whose disease is advanced and associated with a significant deterioration in functional status. These patients are bed-bound and unable to perform various tasks of self-care such as dressing and washing. Another group consists of individuals in the final phase of an irreversible decline who are manifesting the anorexia-cachexia syndrome of rapidly progressive tumors. These patients have severe malnutrition and a life expectancy of less than two months.

Dissimilarities Between PCU and Other Conditions

According to James Hoeffler, there are some conditions that could warrant forgoing ANH. Among them: terminal illness, irreversible unconsciousness, and severe dementia.[35] Should PCU be added to this list?

There appear to be some medical facts about PCU that make

it distinct. First, in PCU, the onset of the disorder is sudden. It results from an initial period of coma caused by trauma, drug overdose, anoxia, severe stroke or infection. In this context, initial resuscitation usually occurs in an intensive care unit where a number of life-sustaining technologies are employed. Given the diagnostic and prognostic uncertainties, ANH is usually initiated along with other resuscitative and life-supporting measures.

A second distinctive feature of PCU is that the majority of patients who suffer from it are relatively young (i.e., less than 60 years old). They are otherwise physically healthy, do not have a progressive underlying condition, and are not close to death as long as they are supported by ANH. In fact, the most common causes of death among young adults in the developed world are trauma (usually as a result of motor-vehicle accidents) and suicides. Many of these young people will undergo resuscitative attempts that sometimes will leave them in a PCU.

A third distinctive feature of PCU is that patients apparently "progress" from a coma to being wakeful but unaware. It is a progression that raises hopes of still further improvement with time. PCU is also a condition in which one is unable to reject entirely the possibility of some future improvement, even if improvement means that the patient may be left with significant disabilities.

Given this constellation of somewhat singular features characteristic of PCU, can one simply transfer ethical judgements about providing ANH to patients with more common conditions such as severe dementia, terminal illness or permanent unconsciousness to patients with PCU? To answer this question, I will compare various conditions with PCU in light of whether ANH is likely: (a) to preserve life; (b) decrease suffering; or (c) be superior to alternative options.

Does ANH Preserve Life?

People with PCU are unable to swallow food or fluids. Although they may swallow spontaneously, this does not mean that they are able to eat or drink. Trying to provide nutrition orally in these cases would be like trying to feed someone who is asleep or deeply sedated. Without nutrition and hydration provided to them by means other than oral feeding, people with PCU will die of dehydration in a matter of a few days or, at most, one or two weeks.

Similar levels of impaired consciousness might occur in infants with anencephaly, in individuals with a severe stroke, or those with cancer who develop delirium. In each of these conditions, if ANH is provided, patients will survive longer than without ANH. Without ANH, certain death will follow within a short period of time (i.e., less than two weeks).

By contrast, for patients with other conditions, ANH may not be used to make the difference between life and death. Patients in the last stages of terminal cancer or suffering from Alzheimer's Disease may be capable of ingesting some food and fluids by mouth. In such cases, ANH may be used to supplement or optimize impaired nutrition or to make the feeding process more time efficient for caregivers, rather than to preserve life. Similarly, in conditions such as stroke and Parkinson's Disease, ANH might be used to minimize risks due to dysphagia, such as choking or aspirating food or fluids into the lungs. Even in these instances, some oral intake of food and fluids may be possible unless there is impaired consciousness, severe swallowing difficulties, or an oral-pharyngeal cancer that obstructs the gastrointestinal tract.

Does ANH Relieve Suffering?

It is sometimes supposed that individuals with impaired consciousness, to the extent that they have no awareness, may nevertheless experience pain at some level. Since intact cerebral hemispheric functioning is necessary in order to perceive pain, those whose brain functions are restricted to the brain stem level cannot be said to "experience" pain or to suffer physically or mentally. They cannot experience thirst or hunger. Attention to hunger and thirst, however, is relevant for individuals who are unable to ingest food or fluids by mouth and who are sufficiently aware that they might experience the deprivation associated with forgoing nutrition and hydration. These might include patients suffering from conditions such as stroke, Parkinson's Disease, ALS, dementia, and obstructing cancers of the oral-pharynx or esophagus.

Some argue that, although people in PCU are assumed not to be able to experience pain, other factors such as distress or financial burden to family members and the health care system ought to be considered morally relevant when deciding about ANH.

Is ANH Superior to Alternative Approaches?

Any decision about ANH must not be limited to a calculation of the benefits and burdens of providing or not providing the intervention; it must also take into account the alternatives that might exist to ANH. There are, for instance, a variety of methods of providing ANH that might mitigate particular distressing symptoms (e.g., avoiding nasogastric tubes in demented patients). The decision not to provide ANH does not mean that the patient is to be abandoned. Other concrete alternatives to ANH should also be considered, including hand-feeding if possible. Mouth and skin care, medications to assuage thirst and hunger and control pain, and emotional and spiritual support should continue to be provided as needed. Finally, "benefits" and "burdens" refer to particular, concrete goods for particular individuals and contexts. Sometimes it may be necessary to try a particular intervention in order to obtain an accurate assessment of its benefits and burdens.

Implications for Care

In general, health care workers are likely to support forgoing ANH for those patients with: (1) very low functional status and little or no chance of improvement (e.g., end-stage dementia); (2) a short life expectancy even with ANH (i.e., days or weeks); and (3) discomfort as a result of ANH (e.g., precipitating shortness of breath or uncomfortable swelling of tissues). In such cases, symptom management, although important throughout the course of treatment, becomes an increasing priority of care as life expectancy and functional status decline.[36]

What happens when the goals of enhancing function conflict with those of providing comfort? This question is currently at the heart of a debate in the palliative care literature. Artificial hydration is provided to dying patients in an effort to improve cognitive functioning by correcting delirium. But should it be used for patients who are sedated at the end of life and so are unable to take fluids orally? Ashby, a palliative care physician, believes that providing hydration does not contribute to the patient's comfort or quality of life and would only be an attempt to treat transiently reversible components of an overall dying process.[37] Summarizing the empirical evidence related to the use of ANH in terminally ill patients, Winter supports Ashby's view that hydration "may increase suffering without improving outcome."[38] It has been observed that hydration is not essential for the comfort of dying patients. Furthermore, changes brought about as a result of dehydration, such as hypernatremia, can lead to a clouding of the patient's sensorium and eventually to a coma, a condition that would eliminate experiences of thirst, hunger or other discomforts. In many palliative care settings, artificial hydration is not part of the usual care of such patients.[39]

On the other side of this debate, some have argued for hydration as a basic component in the care of those terminally ill patients who are being sedated for intractable pain but are not evidently in their last days of life. Craig argues that, even when death is inevitable, the benefit/burden calculus favours providing hydration, particularly when the concerns of family are taken into account along with those of the patient. Hydration can be provided easily, is adjusted to the appropriate rate to avoid the risks of over-hydration, and may reassure all concerned that the patient is dying of his or her disease rather than the sedating medications that have led to dehydration.[40]

In trying to determine the importance of hydration in patients with advanced cancer, Lawlor et al. conducted a prospective study of 104 such patients to determine the incidence and reversibility of delirium, a neuropsychiatric condition that impedes attention and communication, thereby contributing to distress. Lawlor et al. found that delirium occurs in 88% of such patients. It usually occurs not in the final stages of the dying process, but some sixteen days before death. Delirium was found to be an independent predictor of poor survival and to be reversible in approximately 50% of cases. The causes of delirium were multi-factorial, and its reversal was effected by minimally invasive measures such as discontinuing or reducing the dose of certain medications and by hydrating patients.[41]

There are, therefore, opposing views on the topic of hydrating the terminally ill close to death. For some, dehydration and the resulting delirium are considered to be a normal physiological aspect of dying. For others, delirium is a pathological process that undermines the quality of life of patients in the terminal stages of advanced cancers, which can and should be addressed by hydration and other measures.

A recent study suggests that patients and physicians have very different views on this issue. With regard to factors considered important at the end of life, for instance, patients consistently consider "being mentally aware" at the end of life important more often than physicians do (92% to 65% of those surveyed). This suggests that patients are more likely than physicians to support the enhancement of cognitive functioning at the end of life over efforts to control symptoms if the two are in conflict.[42]

Questions

Given these considerations, the following questions seem vital to consider:

1. Are there conditions that are sufficiently similar to PCU that ANH could be considered an "ordinary means" of providing nourishment?
2. Are there conditions that are sufficiently dissimilar from PCU that ANH could be considered an "extraordinary means" in which its burdens outweigh its benefits compared to other possible alternatives?
3. Are there conditions in which there are other relevant questions that need to be considered before determining whether ANH is or is not morally obligatory?

Technical and Symbolic Aspects of ANH

A basic question to be addressed is: in what sense, if any, can ANH be considered simply a means of care rather than a form of medical treatment? Even if artificial or medical interventions are involved, in what sense are they a "natural" and reasonable means of preserving life? To answer these questions, it would be helpful to examine the devices and substances used to provide nutrition and hydration to patients who are unable to take nutrition and hydration by mouth. It will also be good to be aware of common medical indications and counter-indications for the use of ANH. I will start by reviewing two main categories of ANH, enteral (via the gut) and parenteral nutrition (via any route other than the gut). I will then explore some of the symbolic meanings attached to ANH that may influence judgements about whether it should be considered care or medical treatment.

Enteral Nutrition and Hydration

In many of the conditions discussed, feeding and drinking problems arise because adequate amounts of food cannot be ingested orally. Once ingested, there is usually no problem digesting, absorbing and metabolizing nutrients and water, or excreting waste products via bowels, kidney, and bladder. In these conditions, then, the medical issue is to deliver adequate amounts of appropriate food to the gut. This is done by delivering food via tubes to the upper Gastrointestinal (GI) tract.

Nasogastric and Orogastric Tubes

The most widely available, simple and well-known technique for delivering nutrition and hydration to the upper GI tract is by a *Nasogastric* (NG) tube. Basically, an NG tube is a flexible plastic tube, about the diameter of a small drinking straw, which extends from the nose to the stomach. It is lubricated with a tasteless jelly and passed through a nostril and down the back of the throat. Once the tube is confirmed to be in the stomach, often by an X-ray, it is secured at the nose by tape so that it is not inadvertently advanced or withdrawn.[43] A calculated amount of nutritionally adequate feeding formula, the consistency of milk, is delivered through the NG tube by gravity from a bag suspended above the level of the patient's stomach. These bolus feeds are delivered over about one hour and given three times per day, usually at mealtimes, by attaching a bag of formula to the tube.

Newer NG tubes have a smaller diameter, softer texture and a weighted tip containing mercury that facilitates the passage of the tube through the stomach and into the beginning of the small bowel. This positioning lessens the risk of aspiration as less formula remains in the stomach where it can reflux into the esophagus. The newer small diameter NG tubes use a constant drip mechanism instead of bolus feedings.

NG tubes are generally used only up to a few weeks because they are prone to causing irritation of the nostril and can be dislodged. This may provide sufficient ANH for the majority of patients because most patients require enteral nutrition for a period of one month or less. However, if patients have a high risk of aspiration, NG tubes should be avoided.[44]

Orogastric tubes are inserted through the mouth and into the stomach. They vary in size, but can have the diameter of a rubber garden watering hose. Orogastric tubes were commonly used in emergency departments to "lavage" stomach contents of patients following a drug overdose. Water would be flushed into the stomach via the tube and potentially harmful pills or other substances could be washed out of the stomach and removed by means of this tube (usually by gravity). These tubes can be inserted temporarily into the stomachs of patients and then removed. However, for the delivery of ANH, nasogastric tubes are preferred to orogastric tubes because they are easier to secure and less likely to be disturbed by eating.[45]

Gastrostomy and Jejunostomy Tubes

For longer-term tube feeding, the most commonly used device is the *Percutaneous Endoscopic Gastrostomy* (PEG) tube. A PEG tube is similar to a *Gastrostomy* (G) tube, which was first used on humans in 1875. The PEG tube is inserted through the abdominal wall directly into the stomach using an endoscopic technique first described in 1980. This technique is superior to the surgical technique previously used to insert a G tube because it does not require a general anesthetic. A flexible fiber optic endoscope is inserted into the stomach through the mouth to locate a suitable placement on the inner wall of the stomach. The light of the endoscope marks the spot where a small incision is made on the external wall of the abdomen, which is the site through which the tube is inserted into the stomach. The procedure takes only minutes to complete and is done using sedation (e.g., a short-acting form of valium) and local anesthetic for the skin incision. The tube is sometimes anchored to the inside of the stomach by a plastic disc that secures the tube from accidental extubation.

Compared to inserting an NG tube, the PEG tube procedure carries a greater risk of complications; however, its risks are fewer when compared to those associated with those of the general anesthetic and the surgical procedure used to insert a G tube. The risk of mortality from the PEG tube procedure is 1%-2%. Other major complications from the procedure are not common but include life-threatening infections (1%) and perforation of the bowel (less than 1%). Minor complications include temporary diarrhea and cramping (12%), temporary nausea and vomiting (9%), minor skin infections (4%), correctable blockage or leakage from the tube (4%) and blood loss that does not require a transfusion (1%).[46] Ongoing complications associated with PEG or G tube feeding are similar to those associated with NG tube feeding and include aspiration of the feeding formula, discomfort at the site of the tube, and the need to restrain patients who might inadvertently dislodge or purposely pull the tube out. After about two weeks, a tract of skin is formed around the tube between the abdominal skin and the stomach, in the same way that a tract of skin will form around the metallic stud used in a pierced ear. If the tube is subsequently removed once this tract is formed, it can usually be reinserted directly without the need of another procedure. If the tube is no longer needed, it can be removed and the tract will close over.

As mentioned above, there are no randomized trials comparing similar patients with and without feeding tubes in terms of overall survival. Non-randomized studies of nursing home residents show no difference in the survival of those with a feeding tube compared with those without one. This result, however, does not rule out the possibility that patients who are tube fed have a poorer prognosis to begin with than those who are not tube fed. Case studies indicate that an age older than 85, a prior tendency to aspirate, malnourished status, and a diagnosis of cancer are predictors of a poor outcome even with tube feeding.

An analysis of several studies estimates that 20% of patients with a G tube die within 30 days after placement of the tube, 45% within 6 months and 55% within a year. The data make no differentiation in terms of diagnosis or the health status of patients prior to tube placement.[47]

Similarly, there have been no randomized studies of aspiration in patients with a feeding tube compared with those without. Non-randomized trials suggest that patients who are fed through a G tube are more likely to aspirate than those without a tube. It is not clear, however, if the reason for this is that patients who tend to aspirate are more likely to receive a G tube on the assumption that tube feeding will prevent or reduce aspiration. Case studies demonstrate that 50% of patients who aspirated before placement of a feeding tube continue to aspirate afterwards. Overall, around 16% of patients with a feeding tube aspirate.

A variant of the G tube is the *Jejunostomy* (J) tube. This is a tube that is inserted into the stomach and then advanced into the upper small bowel, beyond the duodenum, and into the jejunum. The advantage of a J tube is that the risks of aspiration are reduced (though not eliminated). The disadvantage is that a more specialized and expensive feeding formula is required and the risks of diarrhea are greater.

In general, enteral routes of administering ANH are less hazardous and expensive than parenteral routes. The location of PEG tubes (either G or J tubes) makes them relatively comfortable and avoids nasal, pharyngeal and esophageal irritation. Since there is less reflux and aspiration with G tubes as compared to NG tubes, overnight feeding is safer, which may be important for mobile patients who do not want to be constrained during the day.[48]

Proctoclysis or Rectal Tubes

Another enteral method for providing ANH to patients that was used historically but is no longer favoured because it is not aesthetically pleasing is proctoclysis or Murphy's drip (1857-1914). This involved the insertion of a rectal tube through which up to 24 liters of fluid per day could be administered by a constant drip enema. Fluids contained appropriate electrolytes, including glucose, salt and sodium bicarbonate. Although these fluids lacked calories needed to sustain nutrition, the fluid would nevertheless be readily absorbed through the mucosa of the large intestine and would maintain hydration.[49]

Enteral Feeding Formulas

While most patients receive commercially prepared feeding formulae, it is possible to deliver blenderized food enterally, that is, food that is made sufficiently liquid to flow through the tube. Blenderized foods are used in many developing countries mainly because they are less expensive than commercially prepared feeding formulae. The simplest method of administering them is by means of an orogastric tube. Patients with digestion and absorption problems, such as lactose intolerance, may need predigested nutrients generally not available in blenderized foods. There is also a risk of food contamination causing gastroenteritis, which is more serious with J tubes. For this reason, blenderized foods are not suitable for jejunal feeding. Jejunal feeds also need to be specially formulated to avoid causing diarrhea.[50]

Parenteral Nutrition and Hydration

Parenteral techniques of providing nutrition and hydration were developed before enteral techniques. The first hypodermic syringe was used by the French surgeon, Pravez, in 1851. Today, the two most commonly used parenteral techniques are *Intravenous* (IV) lines and *Total Parenteral Nutrition* (TPN). *Hypodermoclysis* is also a parenteral means of providing ANH.

Intravenous

First used in the 1890s, IVs supply water, saline, glucose solutions and medications directly into a peripheral vein. The veins used are usually in the arm, although veins in the leg or scalp are sometimes used in infants. A small needle in a plastic canula or angiocatheter is inserted into the vein and then the needle is withdrawn, leaving a plastic canula in place in the vein. IVs can only be maintained for a period of days before the vein becomes infected, blocked or the catheter dislodged, in which cases the IV no longer functions. Moreover the veins of the arms and legs are usually too small to tolerate more concentrated nutrition solutions which contain proteins that would irritate the veins and cause inflammation.

Hypodermoclysis

Hypodermoclysis is a method of providing fluids, glucose, electrolytes and some medications into the extra-vascular space under the skin of the abdomen or thigh. The advantage of this route is that it provides hydration but avoids the difficulties associated with IVs. Fluids and medications can be provided at a slow rate to avoid excessive swelling under the skin and to allow for the slow absorption of this fluid. For this reason, hypodermoclysis has been used in palliative care settings. Although suitable for fluids, as with IVs, the disadvantage of hypodermoclysis is that it is not suitable for delivering sufficient nutrients to sustain individuals. In addition, patients receiving glucose but not adequate nutrition may actually feel more hunger as the glucose suppresses the metabolic processes that produce ketones from fats, which diminishes the sensations of hunger and thirst.

Total Parenteral Nutrition

Total Parenteral Nutrition (TPN) was developed in the late 1960s and became widely applied in the 1970s as an alternative to the IV line for patients who need to be artificially fed over the long term and cannot tolerate enteral feeding. TPN delivers complete nutrition and hydration directly into a large central vein by means of a Hickman catheter which traverses under the skin from a location several centimeters from the site where it enters the vein, thereby minimizing the risk of infection. Heparin is also injected into the catheter between feeds to impede the formation of blood clots in the catheter, which might cause blockages. A Hickman catheter can function for weeks and months, rather than days, as in the case of an IV.

Parenteral Feeding Formulas
Sterile conditions need to be maintained for parenteral techniques in order to avoid serious infections. Moreover the composition of the substances delivered into the vascular system needs to be more exactly formulated than is possible with blenderized foods. Of all forms of ANH, TPN formula is the most expensive. The daily cost of feeds can be up to US$100.[51]

Symbolic Aspects of ANH

Is artificially supplied nutrition and hydration somehow different from other life-sustaining technologies? Is there a symbolic meaning of providing food and water to patients that distinguishes tube feeding from other life-sustaining technologies? On this issue there are divergent views.

In the pediatric literature, many clinicians regard the feeding of children as the "most basic aspect of care". As we have noted earlier, clinicians are uncomfortable forgoing or withdrawing ANH from their pediatric patients.[52] At one time it was considered by many neonatologists and pediatricians to be an appropriate medical judgement to withhold providing ANH or corrective surgery to infants born with Down's Syndrome and an intestinal obstruction known as a duodenal atresia. These infants were allowed to die by dehydration. Such practices are generally regarded now as culpable omissions motivated, not by the perceived futility of ANH or corrective surgery, but by judgements about the quality of life of these individuals. On the other hand, psychiatrists once considered it appropriate to force-feed psychiatric patients who refused to eat, and used restraints and orogastric tubes to this end. Such practices would now be regarded as instances of misguided abuse.

The position statement of the American Medical Association on tube feeding at the end of life may well express the difficulties many physicians seem to have with the attempt to extend the symbolism of basic care to include ANH technologies:

> It is far from evident that providing nutrition through a nasogastric tube to a patient for whom it is unwanted is comparable to the typical human ways of feeding those who are hungry.[53]

The majority of medical and legal thinkers appear to agree that ANH is just another life-sustaining medical technology and, therefore, is optional. Their view is that, like other technologies such as respirators and dialysis machines, ANH needs to be justified in particular cases according to a benefit/burden analysis.

By contrast, some ethicists, such as Daniel Callahan, have argued that there is a social significance attached to nourishing the vulnerable and dependent in our care that makes these interventions very different from other medical acts that involve life-sustaining technologies. For Callahan, the norm of caring for another by providing food and water loses its meaning if the provision of ANH to some individuals is made optional.[54]

If ANH is always obligatory, as he asserts, there are several implications that we need to think through. First, its value would not be dependent upon the receptivity and wishes of the patient. Second, if a given technique, such as TPN, is more effective and feasible than other means of delivering nutrition, a case can be made that it ought to be obligatory (provided that it is available). Many ethicists, however, would not judge that these two implications are reasonable.

Third, there may well be cases in which ANH is at odds with the symbolic importance of providing basic care. For example, does proctoclysis (hydration through a rectal tube) to an unwilling patient convey the same meaning as care? ANH, in all its forms and contexts, may seem analogous to the basic personal care provided by the good Samaritan in the New Testament who did not overlook the man in need on the other side of the road but rather attended to his needs for warmth, food and the cleaning and bandaging of wounds. However, it is possible to interpret the parable in a different way. Some people argue that people can also be abandoned to ANH and other technologies without being cared for humanely.

Finally what limits, if any, are there to an obligation to nourish another who cannot ask for or refuse this care? For instance, if the problem is not merely an inability to swallow but also an inability to metabolize nutrients, as in the case of diabetes, would the provision of insulin not also be obligatory?

Implications for Substitute Decision-Making

Among substitute decision-makers who choose ANH for a demented relative, fewer than half would also choose ANH for themselves if they were in similar circumstances.[55] If substitute decision-makers rarely know what their relatives would have wanted, what is the relevance of this finding? Orthodox Jews consider the provision of ANH for a family member with progressive dementia to be the standard of care. Although several prominent Catholic thinkers do not regard the provision of ANH to patients with advanced dementia as morally obligatory, others do.[56] John Keown is an example of a thinker within the Catholic tradition who argues that the criterion for withholding or withdrawing ANH for any patient should be the value of this intervention for the given patient. In his view, it should not be a judgement about the worth of the life of the patient, whether he or she has PVS, terminal cancer or advanced dementia; otherwise, the decision to withhold or withdraw ANH will be an instance of intentional killing, that is, an omission of an intervention with the intention to bring about the death of the patient.[57]

Questions for Guidelines

The guidelines that we hope to propose on this issue of ANH should be shaped by a horizon of faith. How does a Christian perspective on death mediate these practical matters? In conclusion, I would like to raise some questions that could help focus further discussion of this issue.

1. Are there spiritual considerations about the goals of life, and the related goals of health care, that need to be part of judgements about ANH?
2. What is our understanding of decision-making in health care and substitute decision-making? Are the individual's wishes absolute?
3. If a moral obligation to provide ANH in all cases is affirmed, should the sustainability of this practice in the health care system be ethically relevant?
4. Does the Christian view of a good death preclude dehydration as part of the causal nexus leading to death?

5. Do our philosophical and theological judgements about ANH presuppose a worldview that we ought to examine critically? For example, when we judge that ANH is *always* or *never* obligatory for a person or group of persons, do we assume that such judgements regard the universal rather than the particular, the abstract rather than the concrete, the necessary rather than what is *per accidens*? How valid is this assumption?

Notes

1 Finucane, Thomas E. and Colleen Christmas. 2000. More caution about tube feeding (editorial). *Journal of the American Geriatrics Society* 48 (9): 167-168.

2 John Paul II. 2004. Speech "To the Participants in the International Congress on 'Life-Sustaining Treatments and Vegetative State: Scientific Advances and Ethical Dilemmas'." http://www.vatican.va/holy_father/john_paul_ii/speeches/2004/march/documents/hf_jp-ii_spe_20040320_congress-fiamc_en.html (accessed November 8, 2006).

3 Jennett, Bryan, and Fred Plum. 1972. Persistent vegetative state after brain damage: A syndrome in search of a name. *The Lancet* 299 (7753): 734-7.

4 Vegetative life has the capacity to respond to its environment, as in the case of leaves turning toward sunlight. Such responses are reflexive and not under conscious or voluntary control. Humans, like plants, also have the capacity to respond physiologically and reflexively to stimuli without such responses being under voluntary or conscious control. An example of this is the sweating of palms, flushing of face, quickening of pulse that might occur when one is nervous. The term "autonomic" denotes the independence (i.e., autonomy) of these responses from voluntary control. Although the term Vegetative State is more established in the literature, to avoid the potentially prejudicial implication that such people have become "vegetables", in this paper I will use the term *post-coma unresponsiveness*. This follows the terminology adopted in a draft Information Paper on this condition by Australia's National Health and Medical Research Council, 2003.

5 Australian National Health and Medical Research Council. Information Paper, 2003:6.

6 Hoefler J. Permanent Vegetative State. Available at http://dickinson.edu/endoflife/Glossary. See also Bryan Jennett. *The Vegetative State: Medical Facts, Ethical and Legal Dilemmas* (Cambridge, UK: Cambridge University Press, 2002), 35. The statistics for different countries have a broad range. For instance, in the Netherlands, Jennett estimates the prevalence to be 6.7 PMP. These numbers depend on the extent of the application of critical care medicine, resuscitation, parenteral feeding and infection control, and whether they include cases of advanced dementia.

7 Adams, Raymond D. *Principles of Neurology*. 1977. New York: McGraw-Hill.

8 Jennett, B. 2002, pp. 27-8.

9 Gill, H. 2004. Misdiagnosis of the Vegetative State. Proceedings of the International Congress on Life Sustaining Treatments and the Vegetative State. Rome. Available at http://www.vegetativestate.org.

10 The Multi-Society Task Force on PVS. 1994. Medical Aspects of the Persistent Vegetative State (first of two parts). *New England Journal of Medicine* 330 (21):1499-1508.

11 Jennett, B. and Fred Plum, 1972.

12 Cranford, R. 1996. Misdiagnosing the persistent vegetative state. *British Medical Journal* 313:5-6. Cranford, a member of the Multi-Society Task Force, provides a revealing response to an article by Andrews who reported establishing communication with 17 patients who had been misdiagnosed as being in a PVS. He speculates that "most people would find this condition [severely disabled with paralysis, anarthric, visually impaired, cognitively impaired, and/or feeding tube dependent] far more horrifying than the vegetative state itself, and some might think it an even stronger reason for stopping treatment than complete unconsciousness."

13 John Paul II. 2004. Speech "To the Participants in the International Congress on 'Life-Sustaining Treatments and Vegetative State: Scientific Advances and Ethical Dilemmas' ".

14 Borthwick, C.J. 2004. Permanent vegetative state: usefulness and limits of a prognostic definition. Proceedings of the International Congress on Life Sustaining Treatments and the Vegetative State. Rome. Available at http://www.iospress.metapress.com.

15 Jennett, B. 2002, pp. 39-48.

16 Jennett, B. 2002, p. 47.

17 Sampson-Fang, L., C. Butler, M. O'Donnell. 2003. Effects of gastrostomy feeding in children with cerebral palsy: an AACPCM evidence report. *Developmental Medicine Child Neurology* 45(6): 415-426.

18 Skelly, R. 2002. Are we using percutaneous endoscopy gastrostomy appropriately in the elderly? *Current Opinion in Clinical Nutrition & Metabolic Care* 5(1): 35-42.

19 Angus, F., R. Burakoff. 2003. The percutaneous endoscopic gastrostomy tube: medical and ethical issues in placement. *The American Journal of Gastroenterology* 98(2): 274.

20 Aziz, S. 1999. Neglect and abuse associated with undernutrition in long-term care in North America: causes and solutions. *Journal of Elder Abuse & Neglect* 10 (1-2): 91-117.

21 Mitchell, S.L., J.M. Tetroe, A.M. O'Connor, et al. 1999. *Long Term Feeding Tube Placement in Elderly Patients*. Ottawa: Ottawa Health Research Institute.

22 Elia, M., et al. 2001. Home enteral tube feeding following cerebrovascular accident. *Clinical Nutrition* 20(1):27-30.

23 Skelly, R. 2002. Are we using percutaneous endoscopy gastrostomy appropriately in the elderly? *Current Opinion in Clinical Nutrition and Metabolic Care* 5(1): 35-42.

24 Post, S.G. 2001. Tube feeding and advanced progressive dementia. *Hastings Center Report* 31(1):36-42.

25 Trabucchi, M., A. Bianchetti. 2004. Life sustaining therapies in dementia.

Proceedings of the International Congress on Life Sustaining Treatments and the Vegetative State. Rome. Available at http://www.vegetativestate.org.

26 National Institute of Neurological Disorders and Stroke (NINDS). 2003. Alzheimer's Disease Information Page. National Institutes of Health, Bethesda, MD. Available at http://www.ninds.nih.gov/health_and_medical/disorders/alzheimersdisease_doc.htm (accessed November 8, 2006).

27 Gillick, M. 2000. Rethinking the role of tube feeding in patients with advanced dementia. *New England Journal of Medicine* 342(3):206-11.

28 Mitchell, S.L., D.K. Kiely, L.A. Lipsitz. 1997. The risk factors and impact on survival of feeding tube placement in nursing home residents with severe cognitive impairment. *Archives of Internal Medicine* 157 (46): 327-332.

29 Finucane, Thomas E., Colleen Christmas, and Kathy Travis. 1999. Tube Feeding in Patients with Advanced Dementia: A Review of the Evidence. *JAMA* 282 (14):1365-1370.

30 Major, David. 1986. The Medical Procedures for Providing Food and Water: Indications and Effects. In *By No Extraordinary Means - The Choice to Forgo Life-sustaining Food and Water*, edited by J. Lynn. Bloomington, Indianapolis: Indiana University Press.

31 Note 26 *supra.*

32 Elia, M., et al. 2001. Home enteral tube feeding following cerebrovascular accident. *Clinical Nutrition* 20(1):27-30.

33 Skelly, R. 2002. p. 38.

34 Senft, M., R. Fietkau, et al. 1993. The influence of supportive nutritional therapy via percutaneous endoscopically guided gastrostomy on the quality of life of cancer patients. *Support Care Cancer* Sept.1(5):272-5.

35 Hoefler, James M. 2000. Making decisions about tube feeding for severely demented patients at the end of life: Clinical, legal, and ethical considerations. *Death Studies* 24 (3):233-254.

36 Angus, Floyd, Robert Burakoff. 2003. The percutaneous endoscopic gastrostomy tube: medical and ethical issues in placement. *The American Journal of Gastroenterology* 98 (2):272-277.

37 Ashby, Michael and Brian Stoffell. 1995. Artificial hydration and alimentation at the end of life: A reply to Craig. *Journal of Medical Ethics* 21 (3):135-40.

38 Winter, Stephen M. 2000. Terminal nutrition: Framing the debate for the withdrawal of nutritional support in terminally ill patients. *The American Journal of Medicine* 109 (9):723-726.

39 Phillips, Paddy A., Barbara J. Rolls, John G.G. Ledingham. 1984. Reduced thirst after water deprivation in healthy elderly men. *New England Journal of Medicine* 311:753-759.

40 Craig, Gillian M. 1996. On withholding artificial hydration and nutrition from terminally ill sedated patients. The debate continues. *Journal of Medical Ethics* 22 (3):147-53.

41 Lawlor, Peter G., Bruno Gagnon, et al. 2000. Occurrence, Causes, and Outcomes of Delirium in Patients With Advanced Cancer. *Archives of Internal Medicine* 160 (6):786-794.

42 Steinhauser, Karen E., et al. 2000. Patient/physician differences on factors considered important at the end of life. *JAMA* 284 (19):2476-2482.

43 Major, D. 1986. p. 25.

44 Hoefler, James. "Forms of artificial nutrition and hydration," in *Tube Feeding Options at the End of Life: A Consumer and Caregiver's Guide*, http://www.dickinson.edu/endoflife/ (accessed November 8, 2006).

45 Pearce, C., H. Duncan. 2002. Enteral Feeding. Nasogastric, nasojejunal, percutaneous, endoscopic gastrostomy, or jejunostomy: its indications and limitations. *Postgraduate Medical Journal* 78: 198-204.

46 Mitchell, S.L. 1997. p. 18.

47 Mitchell, S.L. 1997. p. 20.

48 Pearce, C., H. Duncan. 2002. pp. 198-204.

49 Major, D. 1986. p. 23.

50 Pearce, C., H. Duncan. 2002. pp. 198-204.

51 Major, D. 1986. p. 22.

52 Maillet, Julie, et al. 2002. Position of the American Dietetic Association: Ethical and legal issues in nutrition, hydration, and feeding. *Journal of the American Dietetic Association* 102 (5):716-726.

53 Council on Ethical and Judicial Affairs of the AMA. 1992. Decisions near the end of life. *JAMA* 267 (16): 2230-31.

54 Callahan, D. 1983. On feeding the dying. *Hastings Center Report* 13 (5): 22-27.

55 Mitchell, S.L., F.M. Lawson. 1999. Decision-making for long-term tube-feeding in cognitively impaired elderly people. *Canadian Medical Association Journal* 160 (12):1705-1709.

56 Post, S.G. 2001. pp. 36-42.

57 Keown, John. 2003. Medical murder by omission? The law and ethics of withholding and withdrawing treatment and tube feeding. *Clinical Medicine* 3 (5):460-463.

Some Ethical Considerations Concerning Ordinary and Extraordinary Means to Prolong Life

Kevin D. O'Rourke, OP

Introduction

At the request of the Advisory Committee of this conference, this study considers the traditional distinction made in Catholic moral theology between "ordinary" and "extraordinary" means in medicine, often referred to as a distinction between proportionate and disproportionate means. I have also been asked to address the meaning of the terms "terminal illness" and "fatal pathology".

Hence in the course of the presentation I shall consider:

- the difference between euthanasia and allowing to die;
- the moral norms for making a decision to allow oneself or another to die; and
- whether this moral decision may be made only when death is "imminent and inevitable".

Rev. Kevin O'Rourke, OP, JCD, STM, Professor of Bioethics, Neiswanger Institute for Bioethics and Health Policy, Stritch School of Medicine, Loyola University of Chicago, USA.

The Difference between Euthanasia and Allowing to Die

For Christians, and for many others as well, human life is a gift from the Creator, control of which implies stewardship, not absolute autonomy. We are to treat our lives rather like the talents given by the master to his servants, so that there will be a proper return (Mt. 25:14-30). In other words, this gift of life must be protected and used for a good purpose. As precious as human life is, it is not the ultimate or absolute value for Christians; instead we find our meaning and purpose in friendship with God and living with God forever.

The time may come when someone is reasonably convinced that life is coming to an end and a prolongation of life by additional medical treatment is not the best investment the person can make of what time remains. Hence, if further therapy does "not offer a reasonable hope of benefit or imposes an excessive burden" insofar as attaining the purpose of life is concerned, it may be refused.[1] The intention inherent in an act of this nature differs from that of suicide or euthanasia.

Suicide occurs when the intention inherent in the act, the *finis operis* of the human act, is self destruction. Euthanasia occurs when the intention inherent in the human act, the *finis operis*, is to kill another person, and the motive for the act, the *finis operantis,* is to alleviate or remove suffering. To reject additional medical efforts that do not correspond to the actual circumstance of the patient is neither to reject life itself nor the God who gave it, but simply to reject efforts that will not help to complete the purpose of life.

Pope John Paul II explained the distinction between "allowing to die" and "euthanasia" in the following manner:

> Euthanasia must be distinguished from the decision to forego [*sic*] so called "aggressive medical treatment," in other words, medical procedures which no longer correspond to the real situation of the patient, either because they are now disproportionate to any expected results or because they impose an excessive burden on the patient or the patient's family.... To forego [*sic*] extraordinary or disproportionate means is not the equivalent of suicide or euthanasia; it rather expresses acceptance of the human condition in the face of death.[2]

The Moral Norms for Allowing Oneself or Another to Die

In the tradition of Catholic moral theology, the terminology of "ordinary" and "extraordinary" means to prolong life is used to distinguish between medical therapy that must be utilized and medical therapy that may be omitted or removed. In 1980, the Congregation for the Doctrine of the Faith (CDF) suggested that the terms "proportionate" and "disproportionate" be used to make the same distinction.[3] Over the years, these terms have been used by Catholic theologians but have not supplanted the original terms. Hence, in this study we shall use the terms ordinary and extraordinary. However, the use of these terms is far from straightforward, as physicians and ethicists can assign them very different meanings.

As a pioneer in Catholic medical ethics, Fr. Gerald Kelly, S.J., pointed out, physicians use the term "ordinary" to indicate that a medicine or medical procedure is readily available, standard care, and effective. "Extraordinary" refers to medicines or medical procedures that are highly expensive, unavailable, experimental, dangerous, or unproven.[4] From the medical perspective, this designation can be made without reference to a particular patient. Some examples of therapies that at one time were experimental or extraordinary from the medical point of view and which later became standard care, or ordinary, would be blood transfusions and angioplasty.

Ethicists or moral theologians, on the other hand, consider ordinary medicine and medical procedures to be those that are morally required, while extraordinary means are morally optional. The norms by which theologians and ethicists make judgements about ordinary and extraordinary means are thus different from those used by physicians. Typically, physicians adhere to standard practices of medical care. In other words, once a diagnosis has been made, they will look to the accepted methods of therapy for treating a particular disease or illness and, if such methods or means are available, the physician will consider them as ordinary from the medical point of view. At the heart of this is the physician's presupposition that the patient wants to be healed by the means of therapy that might be effective.

For the ethicist or moral theologian, there is no presupposition in an ethical judgement that a "medically indicated" therapy should be utilized. Instead, ethicists and moral theologians will consider the effect that the medicine or medical procedure will have upon the patient, the family, or the community *before* making a judgement as to whether the therapy is ordinary or extraordinary from an ethical point of view. "Will the medical intervention in question offer hope of benefit or will it impose an excessive burden?" is the question the ethicist should ask; not, "Is there a therapy that is medically acceptable?"[5]

Terminal Illness and Fatal Pathology

Let us now examine the terms "terminal illness" and "fatal pathology". According to standard dictionaries, there is little difference in meaning between the two terms. They both signify that there is a disease or illness present in the physiology of a person that will cause death if the disease or illness is not eliminated, circumvented, or attenuated in some way. But the different outlooks of the ethicist and the physician often lead to different and confusing meanings when these terms are used.

Physicians tend to judge the condition of a patient *after* the effects of life support have been established and, if the interventions circumvent or significantly delay death, then physicians will often state that the patient does not have a terminal illness or fatal pathology. This means, then, that the removal or discontinuation of life support is regarded as the cause of death. I suggest that this method of thinking underlies the lower court decisions in the Brophy and Cruzan cases, decisions that were later reversed when the higher Courts determined that there was a terminal illness present, even though its effects had been arrested temporarily. This kind of rationale is evident when physicians state that a person in a permanent vegetative state (PVS) kept alive by assisted hydration and nutrition does not have a terminal illness. Finally, this seems to be the logic behind the recent statement of the World Federation of Catholic Medical Associations.[6]

From the ethical perspective, a terminal illness does not go away if it is merely circumvented or alleviated; it continues to be present after the fatal effects of the pathology have abated. Thus, ethicists will still ask the questions about hope of benefit and degree of burden even if life support is successful in prolonging life. If it seems that the interventions do not offer hope of benefit or if they appear to impose excessive burdens, then the ethicist might suggest that they be removed even though death may follow. In such cases, the death results from the fatal pathology that is no longer abated, rather than by the act of removing life support. While this may seem to be a difficult concept to grasp, in fact it is an application of the moral principle of double effect. The act of removing life support is morally acceptable because its purpose *(finis operis)* is beneficial for the patient. But it has an effect—death of the patient—which one does not will or intend.

As this brief examination of terminal illness or fatal pathology shows, the connotations of the terms must be analyzed and agreed upon well before ethical decisions are made. A potential cause for confusion (regarding the use of the terms ordinary and extraordinary) arises from the fact that the terms are often used as principles, rather than conclusions. To put it another way, from the ethical point of view, no medicine or therapy can be judged *a priori* as an ordinary or extraordinary means until hope of benefit and degree of burden are evaluated for "this patient." Clearly, answering these questions requires a prior, accurate medical diagnosis and prognosis. More than that, it also requires an overall assessment of the patient's physical, spiritual and economic condition. Interventions like surgery, a respirator or tube feeding cannot be judged ordinary or extraordinary for a particular patient unless all the above information is available. Even very expensive forms of therapy must be related to a particular patient before they can be judged ordinary or extraordinary. Ethical judgements concerning ordinary and extraordinary means to prolong life cannot be made in the abstract.

It is often unclear who has the right to make the ethical decision to deem the means to prolong life as ordinary or extraordinary. Clearly, the physician is deeply involved. He or she must present an opinion as to whether the means in question will cure, help appreciably or have no effect on the dying patient. But, as mentioned before, other factors beyond medical effectiveness must be considered. What about expense, pain, and inconvenience? What about the spiritual condition of the patient? Only the patient or the proxy can weigh these factors. Hence the radical right to make the ethical decision concerning means to prolong life belongs to the patient. Pope Pius XII expressed this idea in the following manner:

> The rights and duties of the doctor are correlative to those of the patient. The doctor, in fact, has no separate or independent right where the patient is concerned. In general, he or she can take action only when the patient explicitly or implicitly, directly or indirectly, gives permission.[7]

Consent to treatment and ethical evaluation of means become even more complex when the patient is not capable of decision making and a proxy must make decisions for the patient. Special care must be taken to defend the right to life of such vulnerable patients. It seems that this was the main concern of the recent statement of Pope John Paul II in regard to the care of PVS patients.[8] Should the proxy's task be to express the patient's wishes, that is, exercise substitute judgement, or to determine what would be in the best interest of the patient? In the United States, the legal community has designed the advance directive which seeks to have persons nominate proxies to express their wishes when they are no longer able to make decisions about health care for themselves.

Thus, substitute judgement seems to be favored in most cases insofar as advance directives are concerned. However, in keeping with the admonition of Christ to love our neighbour, it seems that "best interest" should be the norm for proxy decision making, even if such a decision would lead the proxy to act contrary to an advance directive. While this is not the forum to have a debate on the matter, I believe that the legal community in the United States envisions death as a legal, not a spiritual, experience and that autonomy should trump all other interests, even the spiritual, should there be a conflict of opinion.

Hope of Benefit and Degree of Burden Explained

While hope of benefit and degree of burden may appear to be simple terms, their application to clinical cases can be complex. In the following few paragraphs I shall consider some of these complexities. As I have indicated in several articles, Benedict Ashley and I believe that the ultimate benefit one seeks for oneself or for another through medical care, indeed through any care, is the ability to strive for the purpose of life.[9] To put it another way, friendship with God is the ultimate goal of personal life and any assistance offered to others must be undertaken with this in mind.[10] We recognize that personal striving and offers of assistance may be directed to proximate goals that might be educational, economic, medicinal, or otherwise beneficial in nature; however, even these proximate goals are ordered to the ultimate human goal of friendship with God.

In order for a person to strive for friendship with God, he or she must have the potential to perform a human act (*actus humanus*), that is, an act of the intellect and will.[11] We designate such acts as cognitive-affective acts and distinguish them from an act of the body or autonomic nervous system (*actus hominis*). Because persons in a persistent vegetative state do not have the potential to perform human acts, keeping them alive by means of assisted hydration or nutrition, whether the intervention is considered a medical means to prolong life or merely ordinary care, does not offer hope of benefit to such patients. Other writers, basing their evaluation on the conviction that prolonging life in a persistent vegetative state offers "great benefit" to the patient, do not agree with our interpretation.[12]

Trying to determine the degree of burden is similarly a complex undertaking. Most will agree, in accord with the *Ethical and Religious Directives*, that the intervention's burden upon the family and society, as well as upon the patient should be considered.[13] Moreover, most will agree that not only the physical burden, but also the economic, psychological, and spiritual burdens should be evaluated as well. But some will focus only upon the immediate burdens associated with the medical intervention itself and not upon the ensuing burden imposed by utilization of the means in question. Let me illustrate the difference using a real life example.

An athlete, twenty years old, was practising for the pole vault by jumping on a trampoline. In the course of his jumping, he lost his balance and landed on the edge of the trampoline, crushing his third cervical vertebrae. Medical technicians were quickly summoned; within minutes they placed him on a ventilator and then transported him via helicopter to Saint Louis University hospital. He was quickly stabilized and within a few days the neurosurgeons caring for him, in response to his questions communicated by his family, informed him that he would *probably* be paralyzed for life and would need continual respiratory assistance. Within a few days, once again through family assistance, he asked to have the life support removed because he felt that life in such a debilitated condition would be too burdensome for him. The neurosurgeons and the ethics consultant, hoping to change his mind, brought in people in St. Louis who were living normal lives with similar handicaps, all to no avail. Finally, after a few months of counseling and pleading, the medical-ethical team assented to his wishes. They discontinued life support and he died within minutes. Several people thought that a respirator, in itself, was not an extraordinary means to prolong life, and said it would be unethical to remove it. But they were not considering the overall burden imposed by use of the respirator.

This case shows that the decision concerning burden will at times be subjective; many people would have chosen to go on living with the same handicaps faced by the young athlete but, even after much counseling and encouragement, he decided that living in that condition would be too burdensome.

Can the Decision to Remove Life Support Be Made Only When Death Is "imminent and inevitable"?

In the writings of the earliest theologians considering the issue, the decision to use or not use life-prolonging life interventions did not rest solely on whether death was imminent and inevitable.[14] For instance, theologians considered whether one should abandon dangerous occupations such as mining, or move to more salubrious climates in order to prolong life (in both cases the answer was no). As recently as 1980, the "Declaration on Euthanasia" asked the question: "is it necessary to have recourse to all possible remedies?" In answer to this question, the document lists many circumstances in which one might refuse "remedies" and does not seek to limit the refusal of remedies to those cases when death is imminent and inevitable.[15]

Conclusion

When interpreting the teaching of the Church about ordinary and extraordinary means to prolong life, there are several cautions that should be observed. The theology underlying the application of these distinctions requires a nuanced understanding of patient desires and patient care. As medical science furthers the ability to prolong life, the questions we currently face will become even more urgent as we ask what is true hope of benefit, and what constitutes excessive burden.

Notes

1 United States Conference of Catholic Bishops, *Ethical and Religious Directives for Catholic Health Care Services*, 4th ed. (Washington: United States Conference of Catholic Bishops, Inc., 2001), nos. 56-57, p. 31.

2 Pope John Paul II, "*Evangelium Vitae,*" *Gospel of Life* (Sherbrooke, PQ: Mediaspaul, 1995), n. 65, p. 117.

3 Congregation for the Doctrine of the Faith, "Declaration on Euthanasia," *Origins*, June 26, 1980. Also Benedict Ashley O.P. and Kevin O'Rourke O.P., *Health Care Ethics*, 4th ed. (Washington, DC: Georgetown University Press, 1997), 420.

4 Gerald Kelly, SJ, "The Duty to Prolong Life," *Theological Studies* 12 (1951):550-556.

5 Edmund D. Pellegrino and David C. Thomasma, "What is Medicine?" in *A Philosophical Basis for Medical Practice* (New York: Oxford University Press, 1981), 58-81.

6 cf. Statement of the World Federation of Catholic Medical Associations, "Considerations on the Scientific and Ethical Problems Related to Vegetative State," *National Catholic Bioethics Quarterly* 4:3 (Autumn 2004): 579-581, n. 4. VS patients cannot in any way be considered terminal patients since their condition

can be stable and enduring.

7 Pope Pius XII, "The Prolongation of Life," *The Pope Speaks* 4 (1957): 393-98.

8 Pope John Paul II, "To the Participants in the International Congress on 'Life Sustaining Treatments and the Vegetative State: Scientific Advances and Ethical Dilemmas'," *Catholic News Service* March 20, 2004.

9 See Benedict Ashley O.P. and Kevin O'Rourke O.P., "Reflections on the Papal Allocution Concerning Care for PVS Patients," in *Christian Bioethics* 12:83-89 and "The Catholic Tradition on Forgoing Life Support," *National Catholic Bioethics Quarterly* Autumn 2005.

10 cf. St. Thomas Aquinas, *Summa Theologiae* II - II, Q3:1. See also *Catechism of the Catholic Church* #356.

11 The material in this section, especially the distinction between *actus humanus* and *actus hominis* is derived from the thought of St. Thomas Aquinas, *Summa Theologiae*, I-II, Q 1, a.1; Q 5, a.1.

12 Germain Grisez, *Living a Christian Life*, vol. 2, (Quincy, Il: Franciscan Press, 1993): 532-34. "Should Nutrition and Hydration be provided to Permanently Comatose and other Mentally Disabled Patients," *Linacre Quarterly* 57, no. 2 (1990): 30-38. Joseph Boyle, "A case for sometimes tube-feeding patients in persistent vegetative state," in *Euthanasia Examined*, ed. J. Keown (Cambridge: Cambridge University Press, 1995), 189-99.

13 United States Conference of Catholic Bishops, *Ethical and Religious Directives for Catholic Health Care Services*, 4th ed. (Washington: United States Conference of Catholic Bishops, Inc., 2001), nos.56-57, p. 31.

14 Pontifical Council for Pastoral Assistance to Health Care Workers, *Charter for Health Care Workers* (Boston: St. Paul Books & Media, 1995), n.120, p. 105.

15 Congregation for the Doctrine of the Faith, "Declaration on Euthanasia," in *More Conciliar Documents,* vol. 2, ed. Austin Flannery, O.P. (Newport, N.Y.: Costello Publishing, 1982), 515-16.

Advance Directives and Substitute Decision-Making in Relation to Providing Food and Water

Nicholas Tonti-Filippini

The Contemporary Trend

Cases of withdrawing nutrition and hydration from people on the basis of medical decisions appear to have become frequent in English speaking countries – especially in my own country where, by and large, such decisions are made without legal or other review. Not all such decisions are made on legitimate medical grounds related to the burdensome nature of the delivery of the care provided or its lack of efficacy. Unfortunately, euthanasia by neglect of reasonable care has become more tolerated, but there is some tension about it. To overcome that tension there has been a trend towards encouraging advance directives and substitute decision-making.

The focus of this paper is on a relatively new phenomenon, the withdrawing of nutrition and hydration not as a medical decision, but because the patient previously indicated refusal or a legally appointed representative of the patient is refusing on the patient's behalf. There are potentially many legitimate factors other than medical factors that may bear upon such a decision; however, the

Nicholas Tonti-Filippini, PhD, is a Consultant Ethicist in the Faculty of Medicine and the Department of Philosophy, University of Melbourne, and Lecturer in Bioethics at the John Paul II Institute for Marriage and Family, Melbourne, Australia.

trend seems to be towards factors that do not seem legitimate. Often the grounds for such decisions are judgements that are related to the patient's level of disability rather than anything to do with the nature of the treatment itself. Deciding to withdraw treatment in order to bring about death because the patient has or will have a disability is euthanasia (suicide or homicide).

As well as the inherent dangers of this trend, there are many issues arising for Catholic and pro-life health care providers with respect to being involved in projects decided by substitute decision-makers in which the death of the patient is sought by neglect of ordinary, reasonable care that is not overly burdensome.

This trend elicits several responses:

a) determination of moral and legal limits around forgoing refusal of treatment, and safeguards for substitute decisions and public advocacy of the need for such limits;
b) moral advice to persons completing advance directives concerning their moral responsibility for their own health and for the predicament in which they may be placing their proxy;
c) advice to health care providers about their moral responsibilities in responding to the circumstances of a patient in need of ordinary care, but for whom there is refusal of treatment by a representative of the patient and/or an advance declaration refusing that care.

On 29 May 2003, Justice Morris of the Supreme Court of the Australian State of Victoria handed down a landmark judgement in a case brought by the Public Advocate.[1] The Public Advocate is responsible for protecting the interests of people with disabilities.

There are many cases worldwide that parallel this case, and the details of this case are illuminating for our discussion.

The case involved a woman (known as Mrs BWV) with severe disabilities, including a lack of cognitive capacity as a consequence of a progressive form of dementia (probably Pick's disease). Family members claimed that, before she became unwell, she had told members of her family that, should she ever become so disabled, she would not want medical treatment that would artificially and unnecessarily prolong her life. This claim could not be substantiated.

The Court proceedings were initiated to obtain a definitive ruling on whether artificial nutrition and hydration delivered through a PEG tube (which is surgically inserted in to the stomach) is either:

- "medical treatment" which may be refused, or
- "palliative care" which may not be refused. The definition of "palliative care" in the Act includes "the reasonable provision of food and water."

The Court decided that it was "medical treatment" and could be refused by a guardian or an agent holding an Enduring Medical Power of Attorney on behalf of a person with a disability that prevented him or her from making or expressing a decision.

Judge Morris found that the administration of artificial nutrition and hydration, via a PEG, cannot be regarded as palliative care, where that expression is used in its natural sense. "Such a procedure is, in essence, a procedure to sustain life; it is not a procedure to manage the dying process, so that it results in as little pain and suffering as possible."[2]

It seems very odd that palliative care would be so defined as to exclude sustaining the patient. An effect of the judge's decision is that "palliative care" would be a euphemism for euthanasia.

The Victorian Department of Health has advised that this decision does not affect everyone with a disability, but only those who have previously expressed wishes about their medical treatment. The judge stressed the many safeguards in the Act that protect the interests of people with a disability. They include, most critically, the fact that a guardian or agent can only refuse treatment if there is evidence that persons with a disability would themselves, when fully informed, have considered that the treatment was unwarranted. (Treatment could also be refused if it would cause unreasonable distress.)[3]

Since the decision, there has been a concerted effort to encourage elderly persons, patients with chronic illness, and residents in aged care facilities to appoint people to represent them for medical treatment decisions and to issue statements indicating that they would not want tube feeding.

The Australian Federal Government has funded some of these programs, including one popular program developed by Melbourne's Austin Hospital entitled the Respecting Patients Choices program. This is not, as one might expect from the name, a program to provide a greater range of choices or resources to patients. It is a program whose clear intention is to encourage patients to opt for an advance directive that would bring about death by neglect in the event that they become demented or terminally ill.

The program includes a Statement of Choices form. There is place for patients or residents to write down what they do not want, but the first option is actually already completed and all they need to do is to tick a box. The first "option" is worded:

> If I reach a point where it is reasonably certain that I will not recover my ability to interact meaningfully with myself, my family, friends, and environment, or I am in the terminal stage of an illness:
>
> I want to stop or withhold treatments that might be used to prolong my life (such treatment may include tube feedings, intravenous fluid, respirator/ventilator, or antibiotics). I only want those treatments which provide me with comfort and dignity as part of a palliative care plan.

Many patients in nursing homes would meet this description of being unable to "interact meaningfully with myself, my family, friends, and environment", as would many people cared for in their own homes. Dementia does that. Lack of adequate nutrition also causes mental disability in aging people.

Simply expressed, this directive means: if I suffer from dementia or am terminally ill, starve me and let me die of thirst. And if I get pneumonia, save the antibiotics, let me drown in my own sputum. The prognosis, "terminal stage of an illness," becomes a self-fulfilling prophecy if it means that the person is to be denied sustenance.

My concern, and one that I share with the medical practitioners who drew my attention to the problem, is that, in the option, there is no stipulation that the refusal is to prevent suffering. There is no limit to what might be refused so that ordinary, non-burdensome care is continued.

The Victorian State Parliament, when it legislated to provide for refusal of treatment and enduring power of attorney for medical treatment, recognised that an intention to refuse ordinary, non-burdensome care that is essential to survival is purely and simply an intention to suicide, and withholding such care is indistinguishable from an intent to commit homicide. This was the point of the Parliament specifying the continuance of palliative care and ensuring that it included sustenance. This was the point of specifying that the law in relation to aiding and abetting suicide and homicide remained unchanged by the legislation.[4]

As it is worded, the dissemination of the Statement of Choices document is an advocacy for suicide and homicide by neglect of ordinary reasonable care.

When the Victorian Medical Treatment Act was passed by the Victorian Parliament fourteen years ago, the case that had prompted the need for the legislation was the predicament of Mr John McEwan, a young man with a C3 spinal injury who had been forced to endure mechanical ventilation against his wishes. At the time, the Parliament was careful to exclude the reasonable provision of food and water from what might be refused. For the purposes of the Act, this was not to be considered medical treatment.

The logic at the time was that palliative care involved helping people to live with the dying process, managing pain but maintaining their functions as best as possible, including sustaining them. Palliative care did not mean hastening their death. The expert witnesses to the Parliamentary enquiry emphasized this very forcefully. The point was that burdensome treatments could be refused or withheld, not the ordinary care needed to sustain patients. The Austin Hospital's Respecting Patients Choices program seems to use the phrase "palliative care" very differently.

The Parliament also included in the legislation the requirements that the legislation not be used to aid and abet suicide or to commit homicide. A reasonable belief that a person intends suicide remains a lawful reason to override his or her wishes. The purpose of the legislation, then, was not to facilitate suicide but to allow patients to refuse to be subjected to a treatment that is in some way problematic for them.

The inclusion of food and fluids in the Statement of Choices document would seem to be based on the judgement made in the BWV case. The Austin Hospital program would seem to have taken the judge's decision to include tube and intravenous feedings in general and has applied this to a broad range of people classified by their disability or by their prognosis, not on the basis of the burdensome nature of the treatment offered.

Many people do fear being subjected to unwanted, burdensome medical treatments. But it is another matter to advocate that they opt for being neglected to death. There is a basic level of care and support that is owed to people in a civilised society.

During the BWV case, the Victorian Attorney General argued that the Court should handle the matter under its *parens patriae* jurisdiction which would require case-by-case determination by the Court in like circumstances. Judge Morris rejected that suggestion and clearly intended to make a decision that meant that the artificial provision of nutrition and hydration in general would be held to be a medical treatment and thus refusable by patients and patient representatives. He sought to make a determination that would be a precedent.

In his list of safeguards with respect to refusal of treatment, the judge made no reference to an exception existing for suicidal or homicidal refusal of nutrition and hydration. That the legislation includes reference to the offences of inciting or aiding and abetting suicide,[5] to the right to use reasonable force if there is a reasonable belief that suicide is being attempted[6] and to other laws, such as the homicide laws, and that the Parliament insisted that the operation of these provisions of the existing law remained unchanged, was not included within the judgement. There is, therefore, at least vagueness now in the application of the law in this respect.

The Law Institute of Victoria advised that, following the decision of BWV, there is now greater certainty about a patient's rights to refuse medical treatment and what such treatment comprises. Similarly this certainty extends to the duties of health practitioners in their care of patients. "The health and aged care sectors have an obligation to ensure that policy and practices reflect the understanding of the law as a result of the BWV case."[7]

The Institute made no reference to the responsibilities of health care providers if they have reasonable grounds for believing that the intent of the refusal of care is suicidal on the part of the patient, or homicidal on the part of a representative (albeit with patient pre-agreement).

A problem for Catholic and pro-life health care providers is that following the case:

a) there has been a shift in thinking that supports and encourages advance refusal of ordinary, non-burdensome care in order to bring about death, and
b) such refusals are now to be considered a right protected by law seemingly without regard to their intent.
c) Thus Catholic and pro-life health care providers are likely to find themselves under pressure to become part of suicidal

projects and, in the provision of non-sustaining palliative care, becoming party to aiding and abetting suicide. Where the decision is a substitute decision by a patient representative, that involvement may extend to being a party to homicide.

Magisterial Statements on Making Decisions for Those Who Cannot Decide for Themselves

Pius XII and Patient Representation

The appointment of a person with enduring power of attorney for medical treatment or similar legal provision places that person in a position of acting with the authority of the patient. Pius XII addressed the question of the representation of an incompetent patient in the following way:

> 19. What We say here must be extended to the legal representatives of the person incapable of caring for himself and his affairs: children below the age of reason, the feeble-minded and the insane. These legal representatives authorized by private decision or by public authority have no other rights over the body and life of those they represent than those people would have themselves if they were capable. And they have those rights to the same extent. They cannot, therefore, give the doctor permission to dispose of them outside of those limits.[8]

Very clearly, in this statement, Pope Pius XII envisaged both that which we would now call "an enduring power of attorney (medical)" appointed by the patient while competent (private decision), and that which we would call "a guardian" appointed by the State (public authority). It would seem, therefore, that the concepts of enduring power of attorney and State-appointed guardians with the authority to make decisions concerning the medical treatment of a patient are morally legitimate options in the moral traditions of the Church.

The text also indicates that Pope Pius XII taught that the representatives of the patient have the same rights over the body and life of the patient as the patient would have had. Earlier in the document the Pope wrote:

> 11. ...In a very large number of cases the "interests of the patient" do provide the moral justification of the doctor's conduct. Here again, the question concerns the absolute value of this principle. Does it prove by itself, does it make it evident that what the doctor wants to do conforms to the moral law?
>
> 12. In the first place it must be assumed that, as a private person, the doctor can take no measure or try no course of action without the consent of the patient. The doctor has no other rights or power over the patient than those which the latter gives him, explicitly or implicitly and tacitly. On his side, the patient cannot confer rights he does not possess. In this discussion the decisive point is the moral licitness of the right a patient has to dispose of himself. Here is the moral limit to the doctor's action taken with the consent of the patient.
>
> 13. As for the patient, he is not absolute master of himself, of his body or of his soul. He cannot, therefore, freely dispose of himself as he pleases. Even the reason

> for which he acts is of itself neither sufficient nor determining. The patient is bound to the immanent teleology laid down by nature. He has the right of use, limited by natural finality, of the faculties and powers of his human nature. Because he is a user and not a proprietor, he does not have unlimited power to destroy or mutilate his body and its functions.[9]

In 1957, Pius XII had asserted the ordinary and extraordinary means distinction:

> Normally one is held to use only ordinary means – according to the circumstances of persons, places, times and culture – that is to say, means that do not involve any grave burden for oneself or another. A stricter obligation would be too burdensome for most people and would render the attainment of the higher, more important good too difficult. Life, health, all temporal activities are in fact subordinated to spiritual ends. On the other hand, one is not forbidden to take more than the strictly necessary steps to preserve life and health, as long as one does not fail in some more serious duty.[10]

It would seem, therefore, that Pius XII envisaged a role for a patient representative, but held that the patient, the representative and the doctor are obliged to continue with ordinary means and that a wish of the patient to withhold ordinary means is not a wish that can rightly be granted.

Addressing himself to the proper role of the unconscious patient's family, Pope Pius XII observed:

> The rights and duties of the family depend on the presumed will of the unconscious patient, if he is of age and *sui juris.* [11]

In relation to the family's duty to provide care he wrote:

> Where the proper and independent duty of the family is concerned, they are usually bound to use only ordinary means.[12]

Congregation for the Doctrine of the Faith (1980)

The above teaching of Pope Pius XII about patient representation was referred to by the Congregation for the Doctrine of the Faith in 1980 in the "Declaration on Euthanasia" as retaining its full force.[13] The "Declaration" included statements that defined euthanasia and clarified the ordinary and extraordinary means distinction by reference to the distinction between "proportionate" and "disproportionate" means.

On the question of who is to make a decision the Congregation wrote:

> In the final analysis, it pertains to the conscience either of the sick person, or of those qualified to speak in the sick person's name, or of the doctors, to decide, in the light of moral obligations and of the various aspects of the case. Everyone has the duty to care for his or her own health or to seek such care from others. Those whose task it is to care for the sick must do so conscientiously and administer the remedies that seem necessary or useful.

Who are those who are qualified to speak in the sick person's name? Can a doctor override them? Must a doctor override them if their judgement is clearly indifferent to the needs and interests of the patient or malicious?

A later sentence in the "Declaration" would seem to leave it open as to who makes the judgement:

> In any case, it will be possible to make a correct judgment as to the means by studying the type of treatment to be used, its degree of complexity or risk, its cost and the possibilities of using it, and comparing these elements with the result that can be expected, taking into account the state of the sick person and his or her physical and moral resources.

Pope John Paul II (1995)

In his encyclical, *Evangelium Vitae*, Pope John Paul II affirmed with some clarification the earlier teaching of the Congregation for the Doctrine of the Faith. He writes:

> 65. …Euthanasia must be distinguished from the decision to forego [*sic*] so-called "aggressive medical treatment," in other words, medical procedures which no longer correspond to the real situation of the patient, either because they are by now disproportionate to any expected results or because they impose an excessive burden on the patient and his family. In such situations, when death is clearly imminent and inevitable, one can in conscience "refuse forms of treatment that would only secure a precarious and burdensome prolongation of life, so long as the normal care due to the sick person

> in similar cases is not interrupted". Certainly there is a moral obligation to care for oneself and to allow oneself to be cared for, but this duty must take account of concrete circumstances. It needs to be determined whether the means of treatment available are objectively proportionate to the prospects for improvement. To forego [*sic*] extraordinary or disproportionate means is not the equivalent of suicide or euthanasia; it rather expresses acceptance of the human condition in the face of death.[14]

But the Pope did not, in *Evangelium Vitae,* address the question as to who ultimately may decide whether a treatment is disproportionate or extraordinary.

Pontifical Council for Health Pastoral Care

In 1995, a major difference emerged on the issue of representation, between the teaching of Pope Pius XII and the Pontifical Council for Health Pastoral Care (formerly "for Pastoral Assistance to Health Care Workers") in the *Charter for Health Care Workers*:

> 73. With regard to presumed consent, a distinction must be made between the patient who is in a condition to know and will and one who is not.

In the former, consent cannot be presumed; it must be clear and explicit.

In the latter case, however, the health care worker can, and in extreme situations must, presume the consent to therapeutic interventions, which from his knowledge and in conscience he thinks should be made. If there is a temporary loss of knowing and willing, the health care worker can act in virtue of the principle of therapeutic trust, that is, the original confidence with which the patient entrusted himself to the health care worker. Should there be a permanent loss of knowing and willing, the health care worker can act in virtue of the principle of responsibility for health care, which obliges the health care worker to assume responsibility for the patient's health.

> 74. With regard to the relatives, they should be informed about ordinary interventions, and involved in the decision making when there is question of extraordinary and optional interventions.

There is no scope in the Pontifical Council's document for health care decision-making by those appointed by the patient or by the State. According to the Council, the authority for health care decision-making, when the patient is incompetent, rests with the health care worker in virtue of the "principle of responsibility for health care". The family are to be "informed and involved," but not ultimately responsible. There is no option here of the responsibility having been exercised by the patient in advance or having been entrusted by the patient or a legal process to a representative.

This places the Pontifical Council seemingly at odds with the law in Western democracies. The Council has also not taken into account the matters addressed in relation to patient representation by Pope Pius XII. The Pontifical Council places immense confidence in health care workers in this instance assuming the application of distinctions such as ordinary and extraordinary care and a notion of a moral duty to provide care that distinguishes between what is obligatory and what is morally optional. These may be very large assumptions to make about the health professions in a "culture of death." But, even when there is goodwill, there are questions as to who is the best judge of all the factors that may be involved in deciding whether a treatment is extraordinary or disproportionate. Only the patient really knows the nature of other potentially conflicting personal obligations. Further, many factors in medical treatment are experiential for the patient, and only he or she really knows the nature of the burden of the treatment.

In Kipling's words:

> The toad beneath the harrow knows
> Exactly where each tooth-point goes.
> The butterfly upon the road
> Preaches contentment to that toad.[15]

Presumably a person whom the patient elects to represent him or her may also have a better knowledge of the impact of treatment upon that particular patient and of the patient's circumstances. Does the "principle of responsibility for health care" bind such a person and, if so, in what way?

The Council gives no advice about what precisely the role of the representative is, and what the health professional's obligations are, when there is a person who is a legally appointed representative, such as a person holding a power of attorney for medical treatment or a person appointed to be a guardian.

In recent times, most Western jurisdictions have attempted to qualify the powers of a patient's representative in relation to medical treatment, often by inserting "patient's best interest" clauses and reference to the "patient's previously expressed wishes".

The inclusion of clauses of that nature gives the health professional and other concerned persons the opportunity to question the adequacy of the representation and to seek to have the representation reviewed. Where the representative seems to be acting contrary to the patient's interests, possibly acting for motives that are indifferent or not well-intentioned towards the patient, then it may be that health professionals have an obligation to seek review and perhaps to overrule the representative, especially in urgent circumstances.

We live in different times from Pope Pius XII, and we live with legal structures that seem not to have been addressed by the Pontifical Council. In relation to Pius XII's teachings, it does now seem necessary to qualify the role of representatives. In relation to the Pontifical Council, we cannot ignore the reality that legal and ethical structures for representation in relation to medical treatment decisions exist, and we need principles to guide health professionals in relation to the role of the representatives.

This is particularly the case in the culture of death where the trend towards "quality of life" assessments in relation to care threaten the survival of the disabled and the incompetent.

There have been various statements on these issues by national Bishops' Conferences. It should be noted that Doctrinal declarations may be submitted to a vote of the Bishops gathered at Conference, when it is determined that it is necessary to deal "with new questions and (to act) so that the message of Christ enlightens and guides people's conscience in resolving new problems arising from changes in society" (AS, n. 22). If duly approved, such declarations constitute "authentic Magisterium".[16] In the English-speaking world, there have been three national documents issued with Bishops' Conference approval that provide some direction on the matter of represented decisions about life-sustaining treatment. They include documents approved for publication by the Canadian (1991), US (2001) and Australian Bishops (2001).

Catholic Health Association of Canada

In 1991, the Catholic Health Association of Canada (CHAC) issued its *Health Care Ethics Guide* with the approval of the Permanent Council of the Canadian Conference of Catholic Bishops.[17]

The guideline for competent dying patients states:

> The informed and voluntary decisions of competent persons, in consultation with their care givers and family, should determine whether life-sustaining treatment is to be undertaken or continued. Health care givers are to promote understanding of available treatment options and to facilitate the dying persons' making decisions on their own behalf.

A later guideline states:

> Treatment decisions for the patient/resident are never to include actions that intentionally cause death.

But the guidelines do not deal explicitly with the competent patient who is dying through refusal to accept ordinary, non-burdensome means of sustaining his or her life. It is unclear whether a doctor is obliged to abide by suicidal instructions to withhold treatment. A subsequent guideline states:

> Competent patients/residents are required to seek those measures for preserving life that offer a reasonable hope of benefit and that can be obtained and used

> without excessive pain, expense, or other serious inconvenience.

It may be that the Association intended this to be an obligation binding on their patients/residents, but would this mean that a person who rejected this obligation would be treated without his or her consent?

The CHAC guideline for non-competent patients states:

> When individuals are non-competent, that is, lack adequate decision-making capacity with respect to treatment, every effort is to be made to ensure that the choice of health care treatment is consistent with their known views. Care givers are to take into account the wishes that the patients/residents stated before they became incapacitated, giving due regard to those wishes expressed in writing. When their wishes are not known, family members or substitute decision-makers will act to promote the dying person's best interests.

A subsequent paragraph qualifies this:

> In deciding for non-competent persons whose wishes may not be known, those measures for preserving life that offer a reasonable hope of benefit and that can be obtained and used without excessive pain, expense, or other serious inconvenience, must be provided.

This would seem to imply that where the patient's known wishes were that they did not want measures for preserving life that offer a reasonable hope of benefit and that can be obtained and used without excessive pain, expense, or other serious inconvenience, then those wishes should be met. In other words, past wishes of patients could be taken to legitimise a medical or nursing decision to end their lives by neglect of life-sustaining care that was ordinary and not disproportionate.

In this respect, the CHAC guidelines would seem to be in conflict with guidelines issued ten years later by the US Bishops and also those issued by the Australian Bishops.

The United States Conference of Catholic Bishops

The fourth edition of the United States Conference of Catholic Bishops *Ethical and Religious Directives for Catholic Health Care Services* (2001)[18] includes a directive:

> 59. The free and informed judgment made by a competent adult patient concerning the use or withdrawal of life-sustaining procedures should always be respected and normally complied with, unless it is contrary to Catholic moral teaching.

This would appear to contradict the CHAC position that did not include the latter qualification.

The US Bishops deal with the question of representation:

> 25. Each person may identify in advance a representative to make health care decisions as his or her surrogate in the event that the person loses the capacity to make health care decisions. Decisions by the designated surrogate should be faithful to Catholic moral principles and to the person's intentions and values, or if the person's intentions are unknown, to the person's best

> interests. In the event that an advance directive is not executed, those who are in a position to know best the patient's wishes —usually family members and loved ones – should participate in the treatment decisions for the person who has lost the capacity to make health care decisions.
>
> 26. The free and informed consent of the person or the person's surrogate is required for medical treatments and procedures, except in an emergency situation when consent cannot be obtained and there is no indication that the patient would refuse consent to the treatment.

The directives do not indicate what should happen in the event that the designated surrogate is not faithful to Catholic moral principles, or there is a conflict between Catholic moral principles and the patient's intentions and values. What do the good doctors or nurses do in those circumstances? Do they treat without consent of the representative or in the face of his or her refusal? It would seem from n. 59 (above) that they could override a refusal of life-sustaining procedures if the refusal was contrary to Catholic teaching.

Catholic Health Australia

In 2001, the Australian Catholic Bishops Conference in full session approved for publication a "Code of Ethical Standards for Catholic Health and Aged Care Services in Australia". The document was then published by Catholic Health Australia Inc., the body that represents the Catholic religious institutes engaged in health care in Australia.

In the Australian "Code", the issue of representation and patients' wishes is dealt with in the following way:

Refusal of Treatment

> 1.16 Patients have the moral right to refuse any treatment which they judge to be futile, overly-burdensome or morally unacceptable, and such refusals must be respected. In addition, healthcare practitioners may not override any refusal of treatment by a competent patient who is not mentally disturbed, clinically depressed or suicidal, irrespective of whether or not they agree with the patient's refusal (see also 5.4). There is, however, an obligation to prevent suicide when this is possible.

The qualification with regard to suicide seems particularly relevant to the circumstances where a patient refuses ordinary sustaining care such as the provision of nutrition and hydration. But more on this later.

Unreasonable Requests

> 1.17 Sometimes patients may request a test or treatment or place conditions on their treatment which a health-care professional or facility judges to be unreasonable. Healthcare practitioners should endeavour to explain to the patient why they think the desired test, treatment or conditions are unreasonable, and thus why they are not obliged to comply with the patient's request or, in some cases, undertake further care of the patient. However, if there are medically and ethically sound alternatives, they should offer the patient the opportunity of a second opinion and arrange for the patient to be cared for by another suitable practitioner.

Medical Power of Attorney

> 1.18 Patients should be encouraged to talk with their family, doctors and other relevant people about their hopes for, and fears of, treatment, and to communicate to them their wishes about treatment should a situation arise in which they are unable to make their wishes known. Patients and residents in care should be informed of their right to appoint someone to make decisions on their behalf should a situation arise in which they were unable to do so themselves.

On the question of feeding, the "Code of Ethics" approved by the Australian Bishops Conference states:

> 5.12 Continuing to care for a patient is a fundamental way of respecting and remaining in solidarity with that person. When treatments are withheld or withdrawn because they are therapeutically futile or overly burdensome, other forms of care such as appropriate feeding, hydration and treatment of infection, comfort care and hygiene should be continued. Nutrition and hydration should always be provided to patients unless they cannot be assimilated by a person's body, they do not sustain life, or their only mode of delivery imposes grave burdens on the patient or others. Such burdens to others do not normally arise in developed countries such as Australia.

This statement seemed to go further than the statement by the US Bishops which held that:

> There should be a presumption in favor of providing nutrition and hydration to all patients, including patients

> who require medically assisted nutrition and hydration, as long as this is of sufficient benefit to outweigh the burdens involved to the patient.

However the US Bishops did add the qualification:

> The free and informed judgment made by a competent adult patient concerning the use or withdrawal of life-sustaining procedures should always be respected and normally complied with, unless it is contrary to Catholic moral teaching.

Thus, if it is contrary to Catholic teaching to withhold artificial nutrition and hydration, then the Bishops direct that the patient's judgement may not be complied with.

The Australian statement suggests that the delivery of nutrition and hydration and antibiotics for infection are considered to be "care" and distinct from "treatments" that may normally be open to be refused by patients.

Consistency of U.S. and Australian Statements with Papal Statement, and the Latter with the Ordinary and Extraordinary Means Tradition

These teachings (of the U.S. and Australian Bishops) are consistent with the statement by Pope John Paul II on March 20th 2004, to a medical conference that I attended on Life Sustaining Treatment and the Vegetative State held by the Federation of International Medical Associations (FIAMC).

In the context of discussing PVS the Pope asserted:

> I should like particularly to underline how the administration of water and food, even when provided by artificial means, always represents a *natural means* of preserving life, not a *medical act.* Its use, furthermore, should be considered, in principle, *ordinary and proportionate*, and as such morally obligatory, insofar as and until it is seen to have attained its proper finality, which in the present case consists in providing nourishment to the patient and alleviation of his suffering. [19] [italics in original]

It would appear that the Pope has adopted a meaning that makes a distinction between "care and sustenance" on the one hand and "medical treatment" on the other. Medical treatments aim to be curative, that is to say, they pertain to the discipline of healing.[20] Sustenance is not in that sense medical. There is a tradition that casts the distinction in this way.

Some authors who have written on the subject, among them Dr. Eugene Diamond, explain the apparent contradiction between Assisted Nutrition and Hydration (ANH) as a life-sustaining "medical treatment" (as it is described, for instance, by the Council on Ethical and Judicial Affairs of the American Medical Association in its "Report on Decisions Near the End of Life"[21]) and as a "non-therapeutic" form of care in this way: the insertion of the tube is a medical procedure that requires the skills of a surgeon but it is not therapeutic since the tube is merely a vehicle for introducing food and fluids into the body. Yet food and fluids are not themselves therapeutic and address no pathology.[22] As it was expressed by the Pontifical Academy of Sciences, "there is a strict obligation to continue by all means those measures which are called 'minimal,' which are intended normally and customarily for the maintenance of life..."[23]

"Medical" thus does not refer to something that might only be done by a medically qualified person; rather it refers to the therapeutic or curative goals of the treatment. Some "medical" treatments might be done by non-medically trained people and some care or sustenance that is non-medical in that sense may require medically trained assistance to achieve it.

Judge Morris, of the Supreme Court of the Australian State of Victoria, in finding that the administration of artificial nutrition and hydration is a medical treatment, held that "[i]n my opinion, a medical procedure can generally be described as a procedure that is based upon the science of the diagnosis, treatment or prevention of disease or injury, or of the relief of pain, suffering and discomfort."[24]

This definition, including the words "based upon the science of", is so broad that it would include anything from modern breakfast cereals to almost all contemporary brands of sports shoes, to sports drinks, to calcium-fortified, low-fat milk, to lean beef mince, to luxury car seats, to vehicle safety features, and to Polaroid sun glasses and U/V sunscreens.

The judge also referred to the fact that the substances used for tube feeding, which are also used for oral feeding, are drugs because they can be given in overdose and hence are medical. This makes a bottle of wine a medical treatment and one wonders whether, as a child, the good judge had ever had the experience of eating too much chocolate and the hyperactivity followed by vomiting that it can cause (as a result of the natural occurrence of theobromine in chocolate). Judge Morris' definition just seems to be contrived so as to ensure that sustenance delivered by way of a tube was to be held to be medical treatment.

The crucial matter in whether something is a medical treatment is at least in part whether it is intended to be therapeutic or curative. Sustenance, in that respect, is not medical treatment.

The term "natural" is used, in the passage quoted from the Pope's statement, in its philosophical sense (in accordance with human nature) rather than as the opposite of artificial. What is artificial may therefore be natural, its use being integral to meeting purposes indicated by possessing a human nature.

The Pope's statement that the administration of food and water should be considered, "in principle, ordinary and proportionate, and as such morally obligatory, insofar as and until it is seen to have attained its proper finality", has bothered some who see in this an assertion that no judgement may be made that the means of delivery in a given case could be extraordinary or disproportionately burdensome and that this would challenge the traditional understanding, such as expressed by Don Maurizio Calipari at the Rome meeting, that "the 'ordinary' or 'extraordinary' character of a therapeutic action was a *quality* that can and must be assessed fully not in the abstract but in the concrete circumstances of clinical use, *hic et nunc*, and for a specific patient."[25]

My view is that the Pope has chosen his words carefully. The phrase "in principle" qualifies the assertion of what would otherwise be a statement of an absolute obligation. One may indicate as a general rule, "in principle", as a positive obligation but not intend that the rule be exceptionless. One cannot foresee all possible future scenarios, and hence theoretically there may be circumstances where other principles take precedence.[26] I think that this was the import of the words "in principle" in the papal statement. The Pope's statement thus has a very similar meaning to the US Bishops' "presumption in favour of providing nutrition and hydration".

It also encompasses the "Code of Ethical Standards" approved by the Australian Bishops when the "Code" states:

> Nutrition and hydration should always be provided to patients unless they cannot be assimilated by a person's body, they do not sustain life, or their only mode of delivery imposes grave burdens on the patient or others. Such burdens to others do not normally arise in developed countries such as Australia.

The Pope has settled a long standing debate amongst doctors and theologians concerning whether artificial nutrition and hydration could be withdrawn or withheld when a patient, such as a patient who is in a post coma unresponsive state or so-called persistent vegetative state (PVS), no longer appears to experience a benefit. He is stating that the administration of nutrition and hydration is beneficial if it prolongs life "insofar as and until it is seen to have attained its proper finality, which in the present case consists in providing nourishment to the patient and alleviation of his suffering."

ANH does not nourish if it cannot be assimilated and it does not sustain life if death is so imminent that ANH would not forestall death. If the method of delivery itself imposes a grave burden on the patient and others, then other duties may be more important than that administration.

It is thus consistent with the papal statement and in accordance with the Australian and US Bishops that sustenance including that delivered by artificial means is obligatory, and its withdrawal would be euthanasia and prohibited unless extraordinary factors arise that make the means of delivery overly burdensome or the effort to achieve nourishment unachievable.

Papal Statement also about Human Dignity

By addressing the issue of sustenance in the context of patients in an unresponsive state (PVS) the Pope makes clear that that state does not exclude the benefits of administering ANH. In this respect the Pope is specifically rejecting the view that cognitive disability prevents friendship with God and, hence, that those who lack that cognitive ability do not benefit from the administration of food and water.

After recalling that conference members focussed on the theme of the clinical condition known as the "vegetative state", the Pope affirmed that:

> ...the intrinsic value and the personal dignity of every human being do not change, no matter what the specific circumstances of their life. Human beings, even if they are seriously ill and impaired in the exercise of their highest functions, are and always will be human beings and will never become "vegetables" or "animals". Our sisters and brothers who are in a 'vegetative state' fully preserve their dignity.

It is worth noting in this respect that the Australian National Health and Medical Research Council has recently published a document in which it maintains that the phrase "vegetative state" is prejudicial to the interests of patients who are in a state of unresponsiveness because of illness or brain injury.[27]

The NHMRC prefers the more accurate term "post coma unresponsiveness". Post-coma unresponsiveness (PCU) is applied to patients emerging from coma in an apparently wakeful unconscious state in which there is:

- complete lack of responses that suggest a cognitive component;
- preservation of sleep-wake cycles and cardio-respiratory function, and
- partial or complete preservation of hypothalamic and brain-stem autonomic functions.

The Pope maintained that physicians and health workers, society and the Church have a moral duty toward these persons which they cannot shirk without neglecting the requirements of professional deontology as well as Christian and human solidarity. Sick people in a state of post-coma unresponsiveness, waiting to recover or for a natural end, have the right to basic health care (nutrition, hydration, hygiene, warmth, etc.).

The probability that there is little hope for recovery "when the vegetative state lasts longer than a year, cannot ethically justify abandoning or interrupting basic care, including food and hydration, of a patient." Death by starvation or dehydration carried out "consciously or deliberately is truly euthanasia by omission."

The Pope recalled that:

> the moral principle is well-known, according to which even the simple doubt of being in the presence of a living person already imposes the obligation of full respect and of abstaining from any act that aims at anticipating the person's death....However, it is not

> enough to reaffirm the general principle according to which the value of a man's life cannot be made subordinate to any judgment of its quality expressed by other men; it is necessary to promote the taking of positive actions as a stand against pressures to withdraw hydration and nutrition as a way to put an end to the lives of these patients.

"It is necessary, above all," he added, "to support those families who have had one of their loved ones struck down by this terrible clinical condition. They cannot be left alone with their heavy human, psychological and financial burden." Society must promote "specialized treatment and rehabilitation programmes", "financial support and home assistance for families when patients are moved back home", facilities to accommodate those who cannot be cared for at home, and respite for those families "who are at risk of psychological and moral burn-out." In addition, he said, volunteers can provide "a basic support to enable the family to break out of its isolation and to help it to realise that it is a precious and not a forsaken part of the social fabric."

John Paul II ended by emphasizing, "in these situations spiritual counselling and pastoral aid are particularly important as help for recovering the deepest meaning of an apparently desperate condition."

A feature of the Rome congress was the witness given by so many doctors and nurses engaged in the care of those who, through illness or injury, are no longer responsive. European doctors expressed surprise that, in Australia, doctors and nurses consider it permissible to withdraw basic care such as nutrition and hydration. We were told that in France, where it is not permissible to allow religion to influence medical practice, it is a criminal offence to withdraw food and water from persons in an unresponsive state, even if they have previously requested the withdrawal.

It is a sad reflection on Australia that the Australian National Health and Medical Research Council document on *Post Coma Unresponsiveness* refers to the lack of doctors with experience in the long term care of people in an unresponsive state. Yet, on the corresponding European data, there should be at least 400 Australian patients in that condition. Missing in Australia would seem to be clinics that specialise in caring for people in an unresponsive state, with activities designed to maintain them physically and to stimulate mental capacity.

A major component of the Pope's address is not so much the sustenance issue itself, but a profound statement about human dignity and the fact that human worth is untouched by disability.

The statement by the Pope that "the intrinsic value and the personal dignity of every human being do not change, no matter what the specific circumstances of their life" and that human beings, even if they are seriously ill and impaired in the exercise of their highest functions, are and always will be human beings and will never become "vegetables" or "animals" is consistent with our Tradition.[28]

The Council of Vienna, in 1311, decreed that the parts of our human nature are united together, "namely the human, passable body and the intellectual or rational soul truly of itself and essentially informing the body."

The human being is an inherently rational and spiritual being and does not have several souls - vegetable, animal and intellectual or spiritual. The term "vegetative" should not be applied to human patients, whatever their level of disability, because the term is contrary to human dignity and not a reflection of the reality that the patient has an intellectual spiritual soul.

The polarisation of contemporary discussion of patients who have persistent unresponsiveness represents a clash between modern culture, which insists on "existential" dignity, and the Christian tradition of upholding "essential" or "connatural" dignity.

"Human dignity" has a philosophical and theological meaning that refers to the worth of a human being. The International Human Rights instruments say that every member of the human family has inherent human dignity (it cannot be lost, taken away, given away, sold or exchanged) from which our equal and inalienable rights are derived. This notion of dignity is not dependent on a person's level of function or capacity; each has it simply by being a member of the human family.

But in common parlance we do refer to undignified acts (acts which are not consistent with our being rational beings) and we do refer to undignified circumstances (circumstances that are somehow demeaning to us). The philosopher Herman Speigelberg lists the following attributes of dignity as a concept:

- being both inherent and a goal to be achieved or created and not naturally endowed;
- unassailable but able to be violated;
- independent of recognition but demanded by the disinherited;
- incapable of being lost but lost by doing acts "below human dignity";
- worthy of respect but sometimes linked with respect as in "worthy of respect and dignity."[29]

Much of this, Speigelberg suggests, is explained by distinguishing between human dignity and "treating someone with dignity."[30] He suggests further that "human dignity" may be defined as "the worth of a person who is worth being for his own sake, regardless of his usefulness for another," but then admits that it must be more complicated than that and concludes by saying:

> The search for grounds of human dignity presupposes a full-fledged philosophical anthropology, showing not only man's essential nature, its ingredients, its structure and its place in the cosmos, but also his values, rights and responsibilities.[31]

Human dignity has a philosophical and theological meaning within the Christian Tradition. In *Gaudium et Spes*, the Second Vatican Council taught that the divine image is present in every man and that every man is endowed with a spiritual and immortal soul.[32] It is in this teaching that our Tradition grounds human dignity. Human dignity is inherent; it cannot be lost and is not dependent on capacity. We do not lose our human dignity because we are dependent on others or because disease robs us of the ability to reason and to communicate. Dignity, in the sense of human worth, exists in having an immortal soul, not in an individual's level of functioning. On that basis, loss of function is not itself a reason for not providing life-sustaining treatment.

In discussing the BWV case, Dr John Billings referred to the patient's "undignified and grave incapacity".[33] It is not clear what he meant. His remarks would seem to refer both to her condition (immobility, incontinence of bowel and bladder, total loss of cerebral activity and of cognitive functions) and what is done to manage her condition ("the use of a hoist for showering"). However, it was not claimed that she was experiencing indignity.

The indignity referred to is not the way she feels, but perhaps the way that she would have felt were she to be capable of being aware of her circumstances and what was being done to her as part of her care. Perhaps what is meant is that the relatives feel that her condition is undignified.

Are a competent person's feelings, attitude or desire about such matters, that is, the prospect of degenerating to such a state, legitimate reason to refuse life-sustaining care for the later time? In the patient's declaration, the issue of willing her own death for that later time cannot be avoided. If her declaration is, *do not feed me then because it would keep me alive and I would not want to live in those circumstances*, then this is indistinguishable from a suicidal wish (albeit one for which we might have considerable sympathy). The intention is to bring about death by omitting that which would otherwise have been provided. Given the reason, not wanting to live with a condition that is undignified and lacking capacity, the request is intended to bring about death. The object of the request is to bring about the end of life (of a certain kind). This is to be distinguished from a request that others not undertake a measure that is disproportionate or overly burdensome where the disproportionality concerns the hardship contained in the measure itself.

One can understand the anguish that a person may have over impending loss of function in a degenerative disease, and that a person might not want to burden the lives of his or her family with his or her own self as the illness increases dependency on them. But in considering an advance declaration, it would seem that we are not free to give an instruction that is based on some other notion of human dignity that relativizes dignity to capacity and functions and declare ourselves to be worthless in a given set of circumstances. We may decide that the efforts needed to sustain us impose an undue burden on others, provided that those efforts really are burdensome, and disproportionately so. But the kindness that may motivate us to free others of their responsibility to us is misguided if it involves demanding that we be treated as less than the possessors of the inherent human dignity given to us in our creation by God in his image and likeness.

It was said that, to her family, BWV had been rendered dehumanised and depersonalised by the disease. The wife and mother whom they had always cherished no longer seemed to be there.

Loss of psychological personality often happens as a result of disease, but this is not loss of personality in the sense in which it is important to a Christian, who understands that personality is the result of being made in the image and likeness of God with an immortal soul. That BWV is now unable to respond does not mean that the person has gone. The love that we are called to give is not conditional upon response, but unilateral. The love for mother or spouse is not conditional upon her response. She remains the mother that they had always cherished. While the call upon their love may be greater now because the love receives no reward, the obligation to love remains despite the grave incapacity. More than that, their supportive responses to her needs continue to be virtuous, continue to be the expression of their personalities. Her personhood remains an opportunity for them to develop in the image and likeness of God by loving her, even when she is unresponsive.

Following Christian tradition, Luke Gormally contrasts "connatural dignity" with "existential dignity".[34] "Existential dignity" is the kind of dignity a person acquires in virtue of the character of the choices he makes and which shape his life, and is dependent on a person continuing to function rationally and autonomously. Some authors refer to loss of existential dignity as "becoming a narrative wreck". "Essential" or "connatural" dignity is the dignity that is inherent to a human being because he or she has an intellectual spiritual soul made in the image and likeness of God, is redeemed by Christ and called to communion with Him. It is this notion of dignity that results in us upholding respect for human life from its beginning as an embryo without evident ability to think, throughout all stages, whatever happens, and until the end of life, even though for some the end of life is preceded by a phase of lost intellectual ability.

Making an advance declaration to refuse treatment is thus not without the moral limitation that one ought not ask others to behave in ways which are less than virtuous, to ask them to treat oneself as less than a person with inherent human dignity. A patient's level of disability or lack of existential dignity is not a reason for withdrawing treatment that is not overly burdensome and which would maintain the patient's life.

The problem in the case of the patient who becomes persistently unresponsive is that there are usually no such difficulties once a PEG has been established. The feeding is not itself problematic and it is effective in sustaining life. The "difficulty" is over the fact that the life continues. The moral difficulty over feeding is that the withdrawal of feeding is based on the notion that the life should not continue, which leads to the decision that the feeding should stop. This is the issue that has to be dealt with, not the issue of burdensomeness, or unreasonableness or disproportionality of the feeding. The PEG feeding is obviously none of those things in itself unless some complication develops with the PEG.

Questions are raised about the dignity of what is called "merely bodily life" and with it the issue of dualism - the idea that there can be a bodily human life without a spiritual soul. In other words, when a patient becomes persistently unresponsive, are we any longer dealing with a human life in a meaningful sense? This is a discussion worth having because there has been a medical trend toward declaring permanent loss of consciousness (which is more certain in the case of a degenerative disease than it is in sudden trauma) sufficient reason to believe that there is no longer a living human being, just a body. This would involve a definition of death beyond brain death so as to include permanent loss of consciousness. Many of the ICU units that I have dealt with already practise this even though the legal definition has been loss of all functions of the brain.

If we continue to hold that a diagnosis indicating permanent loss of consciousness is not sufficient reason for declaring that death has occurred, then we are obliged to use ordinary, non-burdensome means of sustaining life, even if the fact that the life continues may itself be a burden to others and may prolong their grief. We are not permitted to withdraw treatment with the object of ending the patient's life. The latter is the unambiguous and constant teaching of the Magisterium.

This issue goes to the heart of the nature of the human person and to the doctrinal rejection of dualism. It is my view that whole brain death can be accepted within Christian teaching because the body is no longer an integrated whole, with integration being an essential characteristic of human individuality. The brain is an essential component, through the neural and endocrine systems, of the functional relatedness of the parts of the body to the whole. Without the brain, there is no longer communication between the parts. But integration remains at least to some extent in a patient who has lower levels of brain function even if the patient has permanently lost cortical function. Moreover, medically, philosophically and theologically we are unable to determine what consciousness is and whether it can be considered to reside exclusively within the observable functioning of the cortex. We must give the anencephalic infant the benefit of the doubt in this respect just as we must give BWV-type patients the benefit of the doubt in that respect. Sustaining a patient is an important part of palliative care. The delivery of nutrition and hydration has great significance since they are a normal part of life without which no one can survive. Their delivery is a basic way in which we show we care for and love one another.

A decision to withdraw treatment or care *because the patient lacks existential dignity* is an omission that has as its object the death of a human being.

In his encyclical, *Evangelium Vitae*, Pope John Paul II affirmed with some clarification the earlier teaching of the Congregation for the Doctrine of the Faith. He writes:

> Euthanasia must be distinguished from the decision to forego [*sic*] so-called "aggressive medical treatment," in other words, medical procedures which no longer correspond to the real situation of the patient, either because they are by now disproportionate to any expected results or because they impose an excessive burden on the patient and his family. In such situations, when death is clearly imminent and inevitable, one can in conscience "refuse forms of treatment that would only secure a precarious and burdensome prolongation of life, so long as the normal care due to the sick person in similar cases is not interrupted." Certainly there is

> a moral obligation to care for oneself and to allow oneself to be cared for, but this duty must take account of concrete circumstances. It needs to be determined whether the means of treatment available are objectively proportionate to the prospects for improvement. To forego [*sic*] extraordinary or disproportionate means is not the equivalent of suicide or euthanasia; it rather expresses acceptance of the human condition in the face of death.[35]

In the Catholic debate there has been a question over whether the statement, "It needs to be determined whether the means of treatment available are objectively proportionate to the prospects for improvement", applies only in the circumstance where death is clearly imminent and inevitable. This passage in the encyclical and a similar passage in the "Declaration on Euthanasia" seem ambiguous in this respect.

The tradition seems clear that treatment may be withdrawn if it is itself disproportionately burdensome or simply futile. Pope Pius XII referred to the legitimacy of withdrawing ventilator support on these grounds without restricting the permission to the circumstances of imminent and inevitable death.[36] The earlier tradition also referred to its not being obligatory to use extraordinary means of care, and this had some meaning when professional health care was beyond what could be afforded by people in ordinary circumstances. Health insurance and public schemes removed some of the meaning from that distinction. Medical care is now within the reach of most if not all people in developed economies. The CDF (in the "Declaration on Euthanasia") in 1980 included "the application of a medical procedure disproportionate to the results that can be expected." But the focus remains on the means, not on a judgement about the worth of the patient.

Careful thinking has also been needed in relation to the use of the word "futile". In this case "futile" means that it would not be effective in prolonging life. Moralists have been careful to explain that this ought not be a decision based upon a judgement that *the quality of life of the patient* is futile or overly burdensome. The decision is to be a decision about the treatment itself, that is, the intervention would not be effective in prolonging life, and not a decision about whether the patient should live or die. Disturbingly, the term "medical futility" has come to be used to describe not the effectiveness of treatment, but the level of disability of the patient. Thus W. Daniel Doty et al. write about "medically futile conditions" in their article in the journal *Clinical Cardiology*.[37] This is different from referring to medically futile treatments.

Medical assistance to prolong life may be obligatory especially where the medical assistance to care in fact reduces the burden of care. This is certainly the case in relation to feeding by Percutaneous Endoscopic Gastrostomy (PEG).

PEGs are most often put in place because they are a much cheaper, much less labour intensive form of feeding than hand feeding a patient who cannot manage to feed himself or herself, particularly if the patient is slow to swallow or has difficulty swallowing. The cost of provisioning and maintaining a PEG is less than 30 per cent of the cost of paying an aide to hand feed.

The emphasis on withdrawing artificial nutrition and hydration (ANH) in this debate is not that ANH is disproportionately burdensome or that it is ineffective. Although some methods of artificial feeding may be overly burdensome (total parenteral nutrition is expensive because of the pathology involved and a naso-gastric tube may be uncomfortable for a conscious patient), in reality, in an unconscious patient, or if a PEG is in place and uncomplicated, feeding is not overly burdensome.

The issue of feeding people who are persistently unresponsive arises because there is a view that they should not survive in a state lacking existential dignity, not because there is likely to be anything wrong with feeding them or the method of feeding. The problem for those who think that a persistently unresponsive patient should be dead is that feeding is effective in maintaining life. The burden is not the feeding but the continued existence.

Issuing an Advance Directive

Determination of Moral Limits for Making an Advance Directive

A person with a chronic, progressive illness, or just of advanced age, may expect to lose the capacity to make and express competent decisions about medical treatment. A declaration in advance may be used to request or to refuse various treatment options.

There are several legitimate reasons why a living will may be important, such as:

- to save one's family from the anguish of making the decisions;
- to ensure future treatment (in a culture of death) that is morally acceptable and consistent with respect for human life and dignity;
- to prevent the over-use of limited health resources;
- to prevent zealous over-treatment.

The difficulty with a declaration in advance is that it only comes into effect when the patient is no longer competent. In making such a declaration one is addressing duties and obligations of others. It would be wrong to make a declaration that requested of them a moral evil or that established a moral obligation that was too onerous.

An advance declaration thus needs to take into account the agent who is to carry out the wish of the patient, the agent's circumstances, the health care team and an objective assessment of the moral goodness of what is requested.

In that respect, an advance declaration ought not be a request for euthanasia defined in our Tradition as an action or an omission which of itself and/or by intention causes death.[38] However, this definition needs careful analysis, especially given that the Tradition also allows for the withholding or withdrawing of means of treatment that are disproportionate to any expected results, or because they impose an excessive burden on the patient and his family disproportionate to the results that can be expected.[39]

In the previous section I discussed this matter in the light of various Magisterial statements including the recent papal statement on the unresponsive state (PVS).

What is clearly excluded is a declaration such as that being promoted, with Australian Government support, in hospitals, aged care facilities and through general practitioners in my own home State of Victoria (referred to in my introduction):

> If I reach a point where it is reasonably certain that I
> will not recover my ability to interact meaningfully with

> myself, my family, friends, and environment, or I am in the terminal stage of an illness:
>
> I want to stop or withhold treatments that might be used to prolong my life (such treatment may include tube feedings, intravenous fluid, respirator/ventilator, or antibiotics). I only want those treatments which provide me with comfort and dignity as part of a palliative care plan.

This is a direction to bring about my death not on the basis of anything to do with the treatments themselves, other than that they would prolong life. The decision is based solely on my being cognitively disabled. It is a rejection of continued existence in a disabled state.

Few would disagree that ultimately it is for the patient to decide, after receiving medical advice, whether or not a particular treatment option is overly burdensome. But that is not what is being encouraged in this case – all treatments that might prolong life are to be refused.

There is no state of disability that makes a person's life of less value. As Pope John Paul II taught in his recent statement:

> Even our brothers and sisters who find themselves in the clinical condition of a "vegetative state" retain their human dignity in all its fullness. The loving gaze of God the Father continues to fall upon them, acknowledging them as his sons and daughters, especially in need of help.

> Medical doctors and health-care personnel, society and the Church have moral duties toward these persons from which they cannot exempt themselves without lessening the demands both of professional ethics and human and Christian solidarity.[40]

It is not a moral option for me to decide that, in a state of disability, even ordinary, not overly burdensome, care is to be withdrawn in order to ensure that I do not continue to live in that state. In respecting my human dignity, there is a minimal level of care that others are obliged to provide and I am not able to remove that responsibility from them.

The trend toward declarations in advance has a negative aspect in that it reflects a lack of acceptance and a desire to control illness and dying. As Pope John Paul II expresses it:

> When he denies or neglects his fundamental relationship to God, man thinks he is his own rule and measure, with the right to demand that society should guarantee him the ways and means of deciding what to do with his life in full and complete autonomy.[41]

Substitute Refusal and Professional Moral Obligations to Provide Ordinary Reasonable Care

There are thus limits on what a patient may refuse in advance. Those same limits apply to those who make decisions on the patient's behalf. They do not have greater rights to dispose of the patient than the patient has.

These decisions must be made on a case-by-case basis. The factors involved in deciding what is or is not ordinary or not overly burdensome care vary from patient to patient and circumstance to circumstance. But there are objective elements to that decision. One of those objective elements is the reality that no patient's life lacks dignity or worth. Each human being is of equal worth whatever his or her level of disability.

There is a need to ensure that health professionals may continue, and indeed ought to continue, to provide the care needed to sustain life where that care is not disproportionate or overly burdensome. There is thus a limit on what can be refused. However, the assessment of burdensomeness of the treatment ought be related to the patient in his or her actual circumstances and his or her personal priorities, including his or her previously expressed wishes.

As a matter of public policy there is a need for agreement on the inherent dignity of every human being, which implies an obligation to accept or provide minimal care to sustain life. This agreement needs to recognise a distinction between intent to die or to kill, on the one hand, and, on the other, the refusal of care that is, in itself, overly burdensome.

The encouragement of advance directives by doctors and health institutions has a sinister aspect because it reduces the legal and ethical responsibility of doctors and health care institutions for their actions. Our experience in Australia is that patients are encouraged to take responsibility for decisions and thus provide a legal or ethical cover for decisions by a doctor, health or aged care institution, or other care provider, that would otherwise be illegal or unethical, even homicidal.

There is a need for public policy to address the vulnerability of patients and aged care residents being offered documentation to complete that removes the obligation to sustain them.

Notes

1 Supreme Court of Victoria, Gardner; re BWV [2003] VSC 173 (29 May 2003) http://www.austlii.edu.au/au/cases/vic/VSC/2003/173.html (accessed November 8, 2006).

2 Ibid.

3 www.health.vic.gov.au/mta/decision.htm.

4 Nicholas Tonti-Filippini, "Some Refusals of Medical Treatment which Changed the Law of Victoria," *Medical Journal of Australia* 157:4 (1992): 277-79.

5 Victorian Crimes Act 1958, s.6B(2).

6 Victorian Crimes Act 1958, s.463B.

7 Advice prepared by Dominique Saunders, Special Counsel and Jennifer Holdstock, Solicitor, Law Institute of Victoria, "Refusal of Medical Treatment," Update – Decision of BWV (http://www.rk.com.au/site/upload/special_update_autumn_2003.pdf), Russell Kennedy Solicitors, 2003 (accessed November 8, 2006).

8 Pope Pius XII "The Moral Limits of Medical Research and Treatment," Address to 1st International Congress on Histopathology of the Nervous System (September 14, 1952).

9 Ibid.

10 Pope Pius XII, "The Morality of Pain Prevention," *Catholic Mind*, v.55 (1957): 260–278.

11 Ibid.

12 Ibid.

13 Congregation for the Doctrine of the Faith, "Declaration on Euthanasia" (May 5, 1980) http://www.vatican.va/roman_curia/congregations/cfaith/documents/rc_con_cfaith_doc_19800505_euthanasia_en.html (accessed on January 12, 2007).

14 Pope John Paul II, *Evangelium Vitae*, 1995, n. 65. http://www.vatican.va/edocs/ENG0141/_PR.HTM (accessed November 8, 2006).

15 Rudyard Kipling, "Pagett, MP", *Departmental Ditties and Other Verses,* 1886, cf. http://whitewolf.newcastle.edu.au/words/authors/K/KiplingRudyard/verse/p2/pagett.html (accessed November 8, 2006).

16 Cardinal Lucas Moreira Neves, O.P., Prefect of the Congregation for Bishops, *Letter to the Presidents of the Episcopal Conferences, Doctrinal Declarations of Episcopal Conferences*, prepared in collaboration with the Secretariat of State, the Congregation for the Doctrine of the Faith, the Congregation for the Oriental Churches and the Pontifical Council for the Interpretation of Legislative Texts. http://www.catholicculture.org/docs/doc_view.cfm?recnum=1136 (accessed November 8, 2006).

17 Catholic Health Association of Canada, *Health Care Ethics Guide* (1991), p. 52.

18 United States Conference of Catholic Bishops, *Ethical and Religious Directives for Catholic Health Care Services*, 2001 http://www.nccbuscc.org/bishops/directives.html (accessed November 8, 2006).

19 John Paul II, "Address to the Participants in the International Congress on 'Life-Sustaining Treatments and Vegetative State: Scientific Advances and Ethical Dilemmas'." March 20, 2004. http://www.vatican.va/holy_father/john_paul_ii/speeches/2004/march/documents/hf_jp-ii_spe_20040320_congress-fiamc_en.html (accessed November 8, 2006).

20 *Collins Dictionary of Medicine* (Harper Collins) 1999.

21 Council on Ethical and Judicial Affairs of the AMA, "Decisions near the end of life," *JAMA* 267:16 (1992) 2229-2233.

22 Eugene Diamond, "Medical Issues When Discontinuing ANH," *Ethics & Medics* 24:9 (1999). Anthony Fisher, OP, "On Not Starving the Unconscious," *New Blackfriars* 74:869 (1993).

23 Pontifical Academy of Sciences, "On the Artificial Preservation of Life," *Origins* (December 5, 1985).

24 Supreme Court of Victoria, Gardner; re BWV [2003] VSC 173 (29 May 2003) no. 75. http://www.austlii.edu.au/au/cases/vic/VSC/2003/173.html (accessed November 8, 2006).

25 Don Maurizio Calipari, "The Principle of Proportionality in Therapy: Foundations and Applications of Criteria", Address to the FIAMC Congress on Life Sustaining Treatment and the Vegetative State (March 2004) http://www.vegetativestate.org/pagina_topics.htm.

26 I am indebted to Ray Campbell for this comment in an email discussion on May 7th 2004.

27 National Health and Medical Research Council (NHMRC), Australia, "Post Coma Unresponsiveness (Vegetative State): A Clinical Framework for Diagnosis," (Canberra, Australia), December 2003. http://www.nhmrc.gov.au/publications/_files/hpr23.pdf.

28 Pope John Paul II, Address "To the Participants in the International Congress on 'Life Sustaining Treatments and the Vegetative State: Scientific Advances and Ethical Dilemmas'." http://www.vatican.va/holy_father/john_paul_ii/speeches/2004/march/documents/hf_jp-ii_spe_20040320_congress-fiamc_en.html (accessed November 8, 2006).

29 Herman Speigelberg, "Human Dignity: A Challenge" in *Human Dignity: This Century and the Next: An Interdisciplinary Inquiry into Human Rights, Technology, War, and the Ideal Society*. Edited by Rubin Gotesky and Ervin Laszlo (New York: Gordon and Breach, 1970) 44.

30 Ibid., 58.

31 Ibid., 61.

32 Second Vatican Council, *Gaudium et Spes* (1965) n. 14, 22, 24. http://www.vatican.va/archive/hist_councils/ii_vatican_council/documents/vat-ii_cons_19651207_gaudium-et-spes_en.html (accessed November 8, 2006).

33 John J. Billings MD "COMMENT: Allowing nature to take its course is not euthanasia" *News Weekly* 3 May 2003.

34 Luke Gormally email correspondence to Dr. Nicholas Tonti-Filippini (December 30, 2003).

35 Pope John Paul II, *Evangelium Vitae, Gospel of Life* (Boston: Pauline Books & Media, 1995) n. 65.

36 See endnote 10.

37 W. Daniel Doty and Robert M. Walker "Medical Futility," *Clinical Cardiology* Vol. 23 (Suppl, II) 2000.

38 Congregation for the Doctrine of the Faith, "Declaration on Euthanasia," repeated in the *Catechism of the Catholic Church* and again in the encyclical *Evangelium Vitae* but with a significant change - discussion follows.

39 Pope John Paul II, *Evangelium Vitae*, n. 65.

40 Pope John Paul II, Address http://www.vatican.va/holy_father/john_paul_ii/speeches/2004/march/documents/hf_jp-ii_spe_20040320_congress-fiamc_en.html (accessed November 8, 2006).

41 Pope John Paul II, *Evangelium Vitae,* n. 64.

Reflections on Artificial Nutrition and Hydration

Colloquium of the Canadian Catholic Bioethics Institute (CCBI)

Context of the "Reflections"

Sometimes, as a result of injury or illness, the elderly lose their ability to swallow and so are unable to receive adequate nourishment orally. When they are in this situation, or when discussing advance directives for health care, the elderly, their families and other care providers need to address the issue of artificial nutrition and hydration (ANH). Decisions about ANH call for good clinical judgment as well as good moral judgment. Such decisions may be difficult to arrive at in a context of uncertainty about present or future factors, or when there is a conflict in the ends being sought, or when the patient has a diminished capacity to make decisions with respect to his or her care.

The Canadian Catholic Bioethics Institute in Toronto hosted a colloquium from June 14–17, 2004, to identify and discuss some issues relating to ANH for the frail elderly and the dying. The aim was to be of service to those who are grappling with decisions or

"Reflections on Artificial Nutrition and Hydration" originally published in *The National Catholic Bioethics Quarterly 4* (Winter 2004), 773-782.

policies about ANH. An important context for this colloquium was the speech made by Pope John Paul II to participants in an international congress on "Life-Sustaining Treatments and Vegetative State" in Rome on March 20, 2004. In his speech, the Pope presented some general moral considerations and addressed a particular medical condition called persistent "vegetative" state (PVS) or post-coma unresponsiveness (PCU). The participants in the Toronto colloquium discussed the significance and implications of the papal speech for intervening in medical conditions affecting the elderly in which ANH is most commonly used. Such conditions include stroke, Alzheimer's disease, Parkinson's disease, and cancers of the head and neck.

The Process of Generating the "Reflections"

The Toronto colloquium followed the general structure of the international colloquium of representatives from Catholic bioethics institutes held last year in Toronto, which resulted in a consensus statement on globalization and end-of-life care.[1] Participants were selected to represent a range of academic backgrounds, experiences, and views relevant to the topic of ANH. The thirty participants in this colloquium on ANH came variously from Canada, the United States, and Australia, and their collective expertise covered the fields of neurology, geriatrics, family medicine, philosophy, theology, pastoral care, clinical ethics, and law. A few participants were commissioned to write papers that identified key issues and controversies in the literature, reviewed alternative stances, and highlighted some focal questions for discussion. These papers by Joseph Boyle, William Sullivan, Kevin O'Rourke, O.P., and Nicholas Tonti-Filippini were circulated to the other participants prior to the colloquium.[2] The colloquium itself took the form of intensive small-group discussions followed, in plenary sessions, by a presentation and discussion of highlights from each group. The small-group discussions focused on a number of real-life clinical cases involving ANH in various medical conditions.

A document written by Barry Brown assembled the most important points raised in these plenary sessions, and brought to light areas of agreement and disagreement. This document was presented on the last day of the colloquium for discussion in small groups and at the plenary session. One representative from each group then worked as part of a team to edit the document, and this version was sent to the participants after the colloquium for a final round of feedback. The process resulted in a statement entitled "Reflections on Artificial Nutrition and Hydration." According to many participants, the most important aspects of this process were the emphasis placed on the daily celebration of the Eucharist and prayer, and the atmosphere of collegiality and mutual respect that allowed for frank discussions.

Overview and Highlights

The "Reflections" do not prescribe what people ought to conclude in every situation where a decision about ANH for an elderly patient needs to be made. Rather the statement draws attention to some moral principles, as well as an approach to making decisions about life-sustaining treatments in the Catholic moral tradition which were affirmed in "Life-Sustaining Treatments."

The pope, in his speech, asserted that ANH "should be considered, in principle, *ordinary* and *proportionate*, and as such morally obligatory insofar as and until it is seen to have attained its proper finality."[3] Paragraph 5 of the "Reflections" offers some points of interpretation of this quotation to which all the participants at the Toronto meeting agreed. Crucial to this interpretation were the words "in principle." Participants took these words to mean that there might be exceptions to the obligation to provide artificial nutrition and hydration when the method of delivery of ANH is "in itself in conflict with other grave responsibilities, or overly burdensome, costly or otherwise complicated" ("Reflections," paragraph 5).

The "Reflections" affirm that every human being has intrinsic value and personal dignity and also that death is a part of the human condition (paragraph 2). Decisions about ANH, therefore, cannot be based on the judgment that persons with a severe cognitive and/or physical disability have less value and dignity than other persons. On the other hand, human life need not always be sustained for as long as possible. This is the basis for the ordinary/extraordinary distinction in Catholic moral reasoning.

A very basic guideline for making decisions about life-sustaining treatments, including ANH, is stated in the "Reflections": "Treatments cannot be classified ahead of time as ordinary or extraordinary," i.e., as morally obligatory or optional. A careful assessment must be made of the benefits and burdens of particular treatments (paragraph 7). In this assessment, a patient's responsibilities in the context of limited financial resources may be a morally relevant consideration (paragraph 9). Another important point is that the ordinary/extraordinary distinction applies to treatments in any stage of an illness, not simply to the time of imminent death (paragraph 8). In some cases, therefore, the withholding or withdrawing of ANH is not an act of euthanasia as defined in the strict sense by *Evangelium vitae*, n. 65 (paragraph 6).

The rest of the "Reflections" deals with two main topics: particular and contingent clinical considerations that may be morally relevant in assessing the benefits and burdens of ANH in medical conditions other than PVS or post-coma unresponsiveness (paragraphs 13–16), and advance directives regarding ANH (paragraphs 17–26). These important topics of concern in the care of the elderly were not addressed specifically in the papal speech.

The "Reflections" point out that the clinical features of medical conditions like stroke, Alzheimer's disease, Parkinson's disease, and cancers of the head and neck differ in important ways from PVS or post-coma unresponsiveness. In each medical condition, various appropriate methods of delivering ANH should be considered in light of the best available evidence concerning their efficacy for attaining desired benefits (paragraph 14). Similarly, in each medical condition, evidence regarding possible risks and burdens that are associated with those methods of ANH must be considered (paragraph 15). The "Reflections" note that the patient and/or family have the main responsibility to make the decision in each case, after considering this evidence in light of personal circumstances. Health care professionals are entitled to give a medical opinion (paragraph 16).

On the topic of advance directives regarding ANH, the "Reflections" acknowledge that there may be cultural and jurisdictional variations in practice (paragraphs 21 and 26). The "Reflections" propose that appointing a representative who knows well the patient's wishes and values is preferable to issuing "instructional directives" about specific types of treatment and care (paragraph 22). The rights and responsibilities of such representatives must be acknowledged (paragraphs 23 and 24). Finally, a patient who formulates advance directives, the representative of the patient who is authorized to make decisions, and health care professionals and institutions that implement these decisions should always respect the patient's inherent value and dignity (paragraphs 18, 19, 20, and 25).

Significance of the "Reflections"

The "Reflections" do not purport to offer a definitive interpretation of the papal speech of March 20, 2004. The participants in the Toronto colloquium propose that what the Pope declared about ANH is not a departure from what is in the Catholic moral tradition concerning the value and dignity of the human person and the moral difference between forgoing extraordinary treatments and euthanasia. The "Reflections" emphasize that understanding and accepting these general moral principles entails that patients, their family, and health care professionals have a responsibility to assess carefully the benefits and burdens of treatment options, including various methods of delivering ANH, in light of the patient's duties. They are also encouraged, whenever possible, to think and talk about end-of-life care. These tasks remain the same with respect to any medical condition and for any patient. Participants in the Toronto colloquium found that discussing particular cases was helpful in two ways: First, participants became aware of contingent factors in each case that were relevant to assessing benefits and burdens. Second, some disagreements that arose when participants were considering concepts and principles abstractly turned out not to be morally significant in concrete cases. An examination of particular cases, therefore, can be a useful starting point for thinking through moral issues. There is a need for carefully considered case commentaries in the bioethics literature.

Not all the signatories of the "Reflections" agreed with every point in the statement. Two topics elaborated in the footnotes of the statement call for further reflection and discussion by Catholic bioethicists. The first issue is whether it is a moral requirement for patients to make decisions about health care in accordance with a deliberate plan for their own lives. A fundamental question here is whether feelings have some role in knowing values and should be considered in these deliberations. The second issue has to do with how to understand a treatment's burdens. Some confine burdens to those of the treatment modality itself, such as pain, suffering, or cost. Others also consider the burdens of the underlying illness. One key question here is what respecting the dignity of persons who are living with a cognitive and/or physical disability entails; that is, whether refusing treatment on the grounds of a present or anticipated detriorationin cognitive and/or physical functioning, whether one's own or another's, is compatible with respect for that person's ontological dignity.

The "Reflections" are the result of an international collaboration. We wish to thank the board and supporters of the Canadian Catholic Bioethics Institute, participants in the Toronto colloquium, and those who helped to prepare and edit this document. Colloquia such as the ones held in Toronto in 2003 and 2004 affirm the fruitfulness of discussions and collaborations among Catholic bioethicists. There is need for similar opportunities for Catholic bioethicists to exchange ideas and to work together in their own countries and internationally. One recent initiative to promote such ongoing collaboration among Catholic bioethicists around the world is being supported under the aegis of various national associations and sponsored by the Sovereign Military Order of Malta. [4]

Reflections on Artificial Nutrition and Hydration

Introduction

1. The Canadian Catholic Bioethics Institute sponsored a meeting in Toronto, June 14–17, 2004. The purpose of this meeting was to discuss the speech made by Pope John Paul II on March 20,

2004 to participants in the International Congress on "Life-Sustaining Treatments and Vegetative State" and to assist health care professionals, patients, their families and the community in making decisions about artificial nutrition and hydration (ANH) for elderly patients who have medical conditions other than a "vegetative state." Participants in the Toronto meeting, who work in various fields related to bioethics and had different starting points and perspectives, agreed that the following reflections summarize generally the outcome of their discussions. Those participants who consented to be listed at the end of these reflections do so in their own name and not on behalf of their institutions. Although all the signatories agreed to the three points of interpretation of the papal speech in paragraph 5, they do not necessarily concur with everything in the reflections.

Presuppositions

2. In keeping with the Catholic moral tradition:

   • Life is a gift from God for which we have stewardship. Illness, suffering and death are part of the human condition.

   • Humans are relational beings who summon a response from others. All human beings, regardless of their state of health or function, are persons endowed with a spiritual soul and created in the image of God. As such, they possess an intrinsic dignity and value, and have moral status. It follows from this understanding that patients in the state known as "persistent vegetative state" (PVS) are persons. It also follows that, even when patients with advanced dementia, such as Alzheimer's disease, have personalities that are diminished, they remain persons throughout the course of their disease leading to death. Individuals with a developmental or physical disability, even in extreme degrees, also are persons with the same dignity and rights as other persons.

"Vegetative State" (Post-Coma Unresponsiveness)

3. The term "vegetative state" was developed in reference to certain functions of the autonomic or "vegetative" nervous system. These functions, such as the regulation of breathing and the heart rate, are retained despite a patient's unawareness of self and environment. Patients in a "vegetative state" have sleep-wake cycles in which they periodically open their eyes, but they show no evidence of response to the environment, purposeful responses to stimuli and language comprehension or expression. Unfortunately some have misunderstood and misused the term "vegetative state" to suggest that persons in this state are less than fully human. To avoid this, it is preferable to designate the condition as a state of "post-coma unresponsiveness".

4. If post-coma unresponsiveness lasts longer than six months following a brain injury from lack of oxygen, or twelve months following a traumatic brain injury, it is conventionally considered to be "permanent." This means that the statistical probability of any recovery is minimal but not unprecedented.

The Papal Speech

5. In the responses to the papal speech of March 20, 2004, there has been uncertainty and speculation in regard to the statement that ANH "should be considered, in principle, *ordinary* and *proportionate*, and as such morally obligatory, insofar as and until it is seen to have attained its proper finality."[5] The meeting reached the following interpretation of this sentence in the papal speech:

• The papal speech needs to be understood in the context of the Catholic tradition. The words "in principle" (n. 4) do not mean "absolute" in the sense of "exceptionless" but allow consideration of other duties that might apply.

• Persons in a state of lost cognitive and affective capacity retain a spiritual soul; their life has intrinsic value and personal dignity, and they must be treated with the full respect and care owed to a human being.

• For unresponsive patients to whom ANH can be delivered without being in itself in conflict with other grave responsibilities, or overly burdensome, costly or otherwise complicated, ANH should be considered ordinary and proportionate and, as such, morally obligatory.

Is Withdrawing ANH from Post-Coma Unresponsive Patients an Act of Euthanasia?

6. *Evangelium vitae* states that:

> *Euthanasia in the strict sense* is understood to be an action or omission which of itself and by intention causes death, with the purpose of eliminating all suffering. 'Euthanasia's terms of reference, therefore, are to be found in the intention of the will and in the methods used.'
>
> Euthanasia must be distinguished from the decision to forego [*sic*] so-called "aggressive medical treatment," in other words, medical procedures which no longer correspond to the real situation of the patient, either because they are by now disproportionate to any expected results or because they impose an excessive burden on the patient and his family." [6]

7. Treatments cannot be classified ahead of time as ordinary or extraordinary. Reference must be made to the wishes[7] and values of the patient, his or her condition, and the availability of health care in the given context. Ordinary measures, in the traditional moral sense, do not involve excessive pain, expense or other burdens.[8] Extraordinary treatments are those that do involve excessive pain, expense or other burdens. The requirement to undertake an assessment of the benefits and burdens is captured in the alternative designation: proportionate or disproportionate. Some treatments may involve burdens that are disproportionate to the benefits; therefore such treatments are not morally obligatory.

8. The ordinary/extraordinary distinction applies to any stage of illness, not simply to imminent death. However, this distinction may be particularly significant when death is imminent, and the person does not respond positively to treatment. In such circumstances, medical responses other than comfort care and pain control are more likely to be deemed extraordinary and thus optional.

9. While recognizing that it is impossible to place monetary value on human life, the cost of treatment can be a morally relevant factor in health care decisions, especially if patients or their families have to bear the entire economic burden.

10. The increasing technological prolongation of life with its high costs should not eclipse basic human care. This is a matter of fundamental distributive justice.

11. While some treatments may be withheld or withdrawn, care should always be provided, and patients should never be abandoned.

12. Helping patients and their families to make responsible

decisions is important. Health care professionals and institutions may be confronted by patients who, with suicidal wishes, refuse ordinary life-sustaining care. Such patients must be treated with concern for their dignity and well-being. Health care professionals should do their best to protect the life and health of the patient while recognizing that there may be legal and professional limits to their ability to intervene.

Methods of ANH

13. The most commonly used methods of ANH include the following: (a) enteral nutrition and hydration through, for example, a nasogastric (NG) tube that is inserted into a nostril, down the throat and into the stomach or a percutaneous endoscopic gastrostomy (PEG) tube that is inserted through the abdominal wall and placed in the stomach with the guidance of an endoscope that is temporarily inserted through the mouth into the stomach; (b) parenteral techniques which include short-term intravenous (IV) feeding by direct infusion into a peripheral vein such as the arm or leg, and longer-term total parenteral nutrition (TPN), in which complete nutrition and water are delivered directly into a large central vein (such as the subclavian). When a condition warrants temporary nutritional support, very small NG tubes that are more easily and safely inserted than a PEG tube can be used.

Benefits and Risks of ANH

14. While raising many principles of universal applicability, the recent papal speech addressed particularly ANH for people in a state of post-coma unresponsiveness. However, in applying these principles to medical conditions from which the frail elderly are far more likely to suffer, such as Alzheimer's disease, Parkinson's disease, cancer and stroke, it is important to note that these conditions differ

in important ways from post-coma unresponsiveness. The benefits of ANH may include improved nutritional status, the prolongation of life, the symbolic value of giving food and drink, relief of symptoms of hunger when these are experienced, preventing aspiration pneumonia, reducing the risk of pressure sores or infections due to poor nutritional status and immobility, improving function, providing comfort, and maintaining human community. Even in those who have a terminal illness, including patients with advanced dementia, some of these benefits may be attainable.

15. The risks or burdens of ANH include, for NG tubes, irritation and discomfort, and the need for restraint when the patient is confused and repeatedly pulls the tube out. PEGs carry risks of complications, such as death, infection, perforation of the bowel, temporary diarrhea and cramping, temporary nausea and vomiting, blockage or leaking from the tube. Paradoxically, some patients for whom PEGs are initiated in the hope of reducing their risk of aspiration may still remain at significant risk of aspiration with the feeding tube. This risk is greater when nutrition is supplied to the stomach rather than the small bowel, given in bolus or single and discrete doses, and the patient is lying down when being fed rather than having his or her head elevated. There may be a need for temporary restraints in some confused patients to prevent the tube from being pulled out. Some restraints may constitute an assault on human dignity and autonomy in persons. Restraints can also lead to complications such as pressure sores.

Is ANH Successful in Patients with Advanced Dementia?

16. Randomized controlled trials are the gold standard in research. There appear to be no randomized controlled trials comparing the efficacy of ANH with oral feeding in patients with advanced dementia. However, there is some evidence from less rigorously

controlled studies that ANH in these patients does not secure any of the benefits listed above. As it would be difficult ethically to conduct randomized controlled trials with patients suffering from advanced dementia, non-randomized studies and case studies may be the only evidence that we can base clinical practice on. Others may find these conclusions debatable. In this situation, the health care professional and the patient's family will have to consider the evidence as best they can. The health care professional is entitled to give an opinion as to the most beneficial and least burdensome type of ANH and course of action.

Advance Directives

17. Advance directives, whether in the form of a written living will (instructional directive) or a durable power of attorney for health care (proxy directive) or both together, are legitimate instruments by which patients may indicate their wishes to accept or refuse a procedure when they are no longer capable of making the decision. Acceptable purposes include:

- to lighten the burden of a patient's family in making the decision;

- to ensure that the future treatment is morally acceptable and consistent with respect for human life and dignity, and the patient's values and culture;

- to take into consideration responsible stewardship of society's health resources;

- to prevent inappropriate or disproportionate treatment.

18. An advance instructional directive must reflect the duty

to respect human life and dignity and to continue ordinary/ proportionate measures.

19. An advance directive must not require another to cooperate in a plan of care that is morally unacceptable to that other person.

20. A Catholic health care professional or institution should not cooperate in implementing a suicidal directive.

21. The requirement of an advance directive by a nursing home or long-term care facility as a condition of admission may be unacceptably coercive. In many cultures, advance directives are not valued, and end-of-life decisions for incompetent patients may be left to family members.

22. For a patient, appointing someone to represent him or her is preferable to issuing an instructional directive, but the representative must be well-instructed in the patient's wishes and values.

23. A person who is a representative of a patient has the same rights and responsibilities as the patient to respect and protect the patient's life and dignity and to authorize care.

24. A health care professional or other caregiver must respect the rights and responsibilities of the representative of an incompetent patient and discuss with the representative the care that is appropriate.

25. A health care professional or other caregiver must seek review of the representation in the event that the representative fails to act in the best interests of the patient, and the patient is endangered.

26. Health care professionals and families need to be aware of jurisdictional differences in custom and law relevant to advance directives.

List of Signatories

Joseph Boyle	Toronto, Canada
Barry Brown	Toronto, Canada
Eoin Connolly	Toronto, Canada
Michael Coughlin	Hamilton, Canada
Paola Diadori	Montréal, Canada
Rory Fisher	Toronto, Canada
John Heng	London, Canada
Christine Jamieson	Montréal, Canada
Nuala Kenny, SC	Halifax, Canada
Hazel Markwell	Toronto, Canada
Moira McQueen	Toronto, Canada
Pat Murphy	Winnipeg, Canada
Patricia Murphy	Toronto, Canada
Fr. Robert O'Brien	Toronto, Canada
Fr. Kevin O'Rourke, OP	Chicago, U.S.A.
John Shea	Toronto, Canada
Fr. Noël Simard	Ottawa, Canada
William Sullivan	Toronto, Canada
Daniel Sulmasy, OFM	New York, U.S.A.
Beverly Tezak	Toronto, Canada
Nicholas Tonti-Filippini	Melbourne, Australia
Michael Vertin	Toronto, Canada
Marissa Zorzitto	Toronto, Canada

July 22, 2004

1 International Colloquium of Catholic Bioethics Institutes, "Globalization and the Culture of Life Consensus Statement," *The National Catholic Bioethics Quarterly* 4.1 (Spring 2004): 151–158. **Editor's note**: Papers presented at the Colloquium were published by CCBI in the collection, *Globalization and the Culture of Life: Proceedings of the Canadian Catholic Bioethics Institute 2003 International Colloquium*, edited by Bridget Campion, PhD, and Leo Walsh, CSB (Toronto: CCBI, 2005).

2 Joseph Boyle, "Towards Ethical Guidelines for the Use of Artificial Nutrition and Hydration"; William Sullivan, "The Role of Artificial Nutrition and Hydration in the Care of the Frail Elderly: Empirical Issues and Disputed Questions"; Kevin O'Rourke, O.P., "Some Ethical Considerations Concerning Ordinary and Extraordinary Means to Prolong Life"; Nicholas Tonti-Filippini, "Advance Directives and Substitute Decision-Making in Relation to Providing Food and Water."

3 John Paul II, Address "To the Participants in the International Congress on 'Life Sustaining Treatments and the Vegetative State: Scientific Advances and Ethical Dilemmas'," March 20, 2004, n. 4 (original emphasis), http://www.vatican.va/holy_father/john_paul_ii/speeches/2004/march/documents/hf_jp-ii_spe_20040320_congress-fiamc_en.html.

4 http://www.iacbweb.org

5 John Paul II, "Life-Sustaining Treatments," n. 4 (original emphasis).

6 John Paul II, *Evangelium vitae* (March 25, 1995; Boston: Pauline Books and Media), n. 65; internal quotation from Congregation for the Doctrine of the Faith, "Declaration on Euthanasia," *Iura et Bona*; May 5, 1980, http://www.vatican.va/roman_curia/congregations/cfaith/documents/rc_con_cfath_doc_19800505_euthanasia_en.html), II.

7 Some participants thought that "wishes" in this sentence should be replaced by "life plan" or some similar term to indicate that such moral decisions ought not be based on whim, but on considerations such as spiritual ends and family obligations.

8 There is considerable controversy over what constitutes burden. Some confine burden to those of the treatment modality itself, such as

pain, suffering, or cost. Others contend that burden will also encompass the conditions of living after the treatment, including being in a state of diminished or minimal consciousness, totally dependent on others, incontinent, paralyzed, etc. Some would argue that these conditions are relevant even if the patient is incapable of experiencing them, as in post-coma consciousness. A distinction can be made between ontological dignity, which all persons regardless of their level of functioning have, and existential or "attributed" dignity, which depends on the circumstances or conditions of living. For some, a diminished existential dignity is an insufficient reason for refusing treatment by advance directive. For others, it is a decisive factor in their reasons for not wanting to live in this state. No consensus was reached on this issue.

Address of John Paul II

"To the Participants in the International Congress on 'Life-Sustaining Treatments and Vegetative State: Scientific Advances and Ethical Dilemmas' "

Saturday, 20 March 2004

Distinguished Ladies and Gentlemen,

1. I cordially greet all of you who took part in the International Congress: *"Life-Sustaining Treatments and Vegetative State: Scientific Advances and Ethical Dilemmas"*. I wish to extend a special greeting to Bishop Elio Sgreccia, Vice-President of the Pontifical Academy for Life, and to Prof. Gian Luigi Gigli, President of the International Federation of Catholic Medical Associations and selfless champion of the fundamental value of life, who has kindly expressed your shared feelings.

This important Congress, organized jointly by the Pontifical Academy for Life and the International Federation of Catholic Medical Associations, is dealing with a very significant issue: *the clinical condition called the "vegetative state"*. The complex scientific, ethical, social and pastoral implications of such a condition require in-depth reflections and a fruitful interdisciplinary dialogue, as evidenced by the intense and carefully structured programme of your work sessions.

2. With deep esteem and sincere hope, the Church encourages the efforts of men and women of science who, sometimes at great sacrifice, daily dedicate their task of study and research to the improvement of the diagnostic, therapeutic, prognostic and rehabilitative possibilities confronting those patients who rely completely on those who care for and assist them. The person in a vegetative state, in fact, shows no evident sign of self-awareness or of awareness of the environment, and seems unable to interact with others or to react to specific stimuli.

Scientists and researchers realize that one must, first of all, arrive at a correct diagnosis, which usually requires prolonged and careful observation in specialized centres, given also the high number of diagnostic errors reported in the literature. Moreover, not a few of these persons, with appropriate treatment and with specific rehabilitation programmes, have been able to emerge from a vegetative state. On the contrary, many others unfortunately remain prisoners of their condition even for long stretches of time and without needing technological support.

In particular, the term *permanent vegetative state* has been coined to indicate the condition of those patients whose "vegetative state" continues for over a year. Actually, there is no different diagnosis that corresponds to such a definition, but only a conventional prognostic judgment, relative to the fact that the recovery of patients, statistically speaking, is ever more difficult as the condition of vegetative state is prolonged in time.

However, we must neither forget nor underestimate that there are well-documented cases of at least partial recovery even after many years; we can thus state that medical science, up until now, is still unable to predict with certainty who among patients in this condition will recover and who will not.

3. Faced with patients in similar clinical conditions, there are some who cast doubt on the persistence of the "human quality" itself, almost as if the adjective "vegetative" (whose use is now solidly established), which symbolically describes a clinical state, could or should be instead applied to the sick as such, actually demeaning their value and personal dignity. In this sense, it must be noted that this term, even when confined to the clinical context, is certainly not the most felicitous when applied to human beings.

In opposition to such trends of thought, I feel the duty to reaffirm strongly that the intrinsic value and personal dignity of every human being do not change, no matter what the concrete circumstances of his or her life. *A man, even if seriously ill or disabled in the exercise of his highest functions, is and always will be a man*, and he will never become a "vegetable" or an "animal".

Even our brothers and sisters who find themselves in the clinical condition of a "vegetative state" retain their human dignity in all its fullness. The loving gaze of God the Father continues to fall upon them, acknowledging them as his sons and daughters, especially in need of help.

4. Medical doctors and health-care personnel, society and the Church have moral duties toward these persons from which they cannot exempt themselves without lessening the demands both of professional ethics and human and Christian solidarity.

The sick person in a vegetative state, awaiting recovery or a natural end, still has the right to basic health care (nutrition, hydration, cleanliness, warmth, etc.), and to the prevention of complications related to his confinement to bed. He also has the right to appropriate rehabilitative care and to be monitored for clinical signs of eventual recovery.

I should like particularly to underline how the administration of water and food, even when provided by artificial means, always represents a *natural means* of preserving life, not a *medical act*. Its use, furthermore, should be considered, in principle, *ordinary* and *proportionate*, and as such morally obligatory, insofar as and until it is seen to have attained its proper finality, which in the present case consists in providing nourishment to the patient and alleviation of his suffering.

The obligation to provide the "normal care due to the sick in such cases" (Congregation for the Doctrine of the Faith, *Iura et Bona*, p. IV) includes, in fact, the use of nutrition and hydration (cf. Pontifical Council "Cor Unum", *Dans le Cadre,* 2, 4, 4; Pontifical Council for Pastoral Assistance to Health Care Workers, *Charter of Health Care Workers*, n. 120). The evaluation of probabilities, founded on waning hopes for recovery when the vegetative state is prolonged beyond a year, cannot ethically justify the cessation or interruption of minimal care for the patient, including nutrition and hydration. Death by starvation or dehydration is, in fact, the only possible outcome as a result of their withdrawal. In this sense it ends up becoming, if done knowingly and willingly, true and proper euthanasia by omission.

In this regard, I recall what I wrote in the Encyclical *Evangelium Vitae*, making it clear that "by *euthanasia in the true and proper sense* must be understood an action or omission which by its very nature and intention brings about death, with the purpose of eliminating all pain"; such an act is always "a *serious violation of the law of God,* since it is the deliberate and morally unacceptable killing of a human person" (n. 65).

Besides, the moral principle is well known, according to which even the simple doubt of being in the presence of a living person already imposes the obligation of full respect and of abstaining from any act that aims at anticipating the person's death.

5. Considerations about the "quality of life", often actually dictated by psychological, social and economic pressures, cannot take precedence over general principles.

First of all, no evaluation of costs can outweigh the value of the fundamental good which we are trying to protect, that of human life. Moreover, to admit that decisions regarding man's life can be based on the external acknowledgment of its quality, is the same as acknowledging that increasing and decreasing levels of quality of life, and therefore of human dignity, can be attributed from an external perspective to any subject, thus introducing into social relations a discriminatory and eugenic principle.

Moreover, it is not possible to rule out *a priori* that the withdrawal of nutrition and hydration, as reported by authoritative studies, is the source of considerable suffering for the sick person, even if we can see only the reactions at the level of the autonomic nervous system or of gestures. Modern clinical neurophysiology and neuro-imaging techniques, in fact, seem to point to the lasting quality in these patients of elementary forms of communication and analysis of stimuli.

6. However, it is not enough to reaffirm the general principle according to which the value of a man's life cannot be made subordinate to any judgment of its quality expressed by other men;

it is necessary to promote the *taking of positive actions* as a stand against pressures to withdraw hydration and nutrition as a way to put an end to the lives of these patients.

It is necessary, above all, *to support those families* who have had one of their loved ones struck down by this terrible clinical condition. They cannot be left alone with their heavy human, psychological and financial burden. Although the care for these patients is not, in general, particularly costly, society must allot sufficient resources for the care of this sort of frailty, by way of bringing about appropriate, concrete initiatives such as, for example, the creation of a network of awakening centres with specialized treatment and rehabilitation programmes; financial support and home assistance for families when patients are moved back home at the end of intensive rehabilitation programmes; the establishment of facilities which can accommodate those cases in which there is no family able to deal with the problem or to provide "breaks" for those families who are at risk of psychological and moral burn-out.

Proper care for these patients and their families should, moreover, include the presence and the witness of a medical doctor and an entire team, who are asked to help the family understand that they are there as allies who are in this struggle with them. The participation of volunteers represents a basic support to enable the family to break out of its isolation and to help it to realize that it is a precious and not a forsaken part of the social fabric.

In these situations, then, spiritual counselling and pastoral aid are particularly important as help for recovering the deepest meaning of an apparently desperate condition.

7. Distinguished Ladies and Gentlemen, in conclusion I exhort you, as men and women of science responsible for the dignity of the medical profession, to guard jealously the principle according to which the true task of medicine is "to cure if possible, always to care".

As a pledge and support of this, your authentic humanitarian mission to give comfort and support to your suffering brothers and sisters, I remind you of the words of Jesus: "Amen, I say to you, whatever you did for one of these least brothers of mine, you did for me" (Mt 25: 40).

In this light, I invoke upon you the assistance of him, whom a meaningful saying of the Church Fathers describes as *Christus medicus*, and in entrusting your work to the protection of Mary, Consoler of the sick and Comforter of the dying, I lovingly bestow on all of you a special Apostolic Blessing.